Healthy Cooking

CANCER PREVEN

COOKBOOK

Healthy Cooking

CANCER PREVENTION COOKBOOK

Paul Morgan

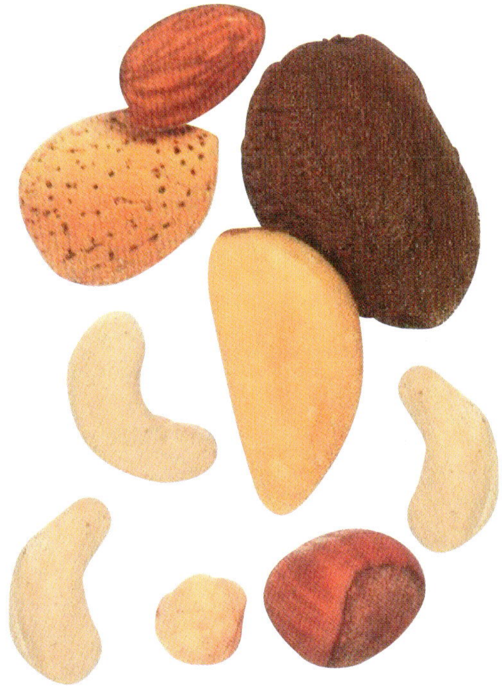

AN OCEANA BOOK

This edition published by Silverdale Books,
an imprint of Bookmart Ltd., in 2006

Bookmart Ltd.
Blaby Road
Wigston
Leicester
LE18 4SE

This edition printed 2006

ISBN 1-84509-230-9

QUMHCCP

Manufactured in Singapore by
Pica Digital Pte. Ltd.
Printed in Singapore by
Star Standard Industries (Pte) Ltd

It is always sensible to consult your doctor before changing your diet regime, but it is essential to do so if you suffer from any medical condition or are taking medication of any kind. If you are concerned about any symptoms that develop after changing your diet, consult your doctor immediately. Information is given without any guarantees on the part of the author and publisher, and they cannot be held responsible for the contents of this book.

CONTENTS

INTRODUCTION

For 25 years or more, theories about what constitutes a healthy diet have chopped and changed. First, all fat was considered to be bad for you – then it was found that some types of fat can protect your heart. Then butter was considered bad, while margarine was thought to be good for you – but after a while, scientists discovered that margarine contained substances called trans fatty acids, which are extremely bad for you. At the same time, all cholesterol was once considered dangerous, but now we know that one type of cholesterol is, in fact, very good for you.

For 17 of these 25 years, scientists tended to mock the insistent claims made by practitioners of fringe and alternative medicine to the effect that people could prevent cancer from developing if they ate the correct diet. But, in 1997, the doubters were proved wrong, when the World Cancer Research Fund and the American Institute for Cancer Research (AICR) published a joint study that was the culmination of 15 years of research: *Food Nutrition and the Prevention of Cancer: A Global Perspective.*

These two quotes from the report sum up both the AICR's position and what is now generally acknowledged to be the indisputable scientific truth:

> *'It is now apparent that though genetic predisposition varies, the key factors determining whether people develop cancer are environmental. The two most important ways to reduce cancer risk are the avoidance of cancer-causing agents, of which tobacco is the most lethal, but which also include biological agents, viruses, and bacteria, and the habitual consumption of diets high in those foods and drinks that protect against cancer'.*

and

> *'The panel found that . . . inappropriate diets cause around one-third of all cancer deaths . . . [it] estimates that 30 to 40 per cent of cancer cases throughout the world are preventable by feasible dietary means'.*

This book will show you how to reduce the risk of developing cancer through choosing a healthy diet, rich in chemicals that prevent the formation of cancer-causing substances and suppress cancer if it does develop. Next, you can choose from a range of mouth-watering, healthy recipes. It may be a cliché, but like many clichés it is true: when it comes to your health, you really are what you eat!

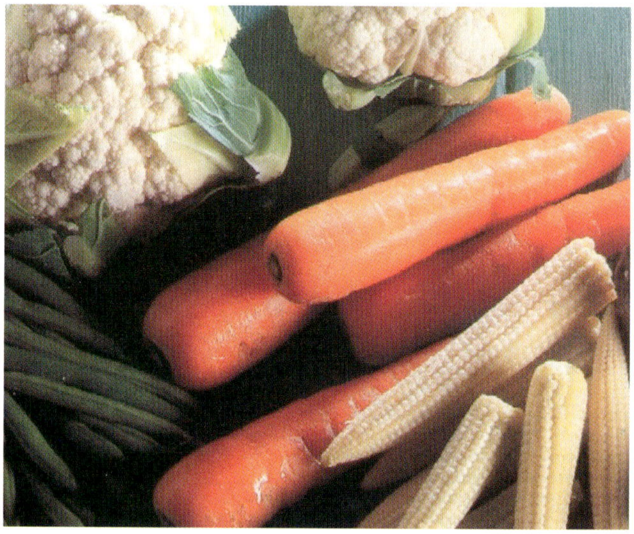

A diet high in fresh vegetables and fruit, and low in salt, will help prevent many cancers.

A LITTLE OF WHAT YOU FANCY . . .

. . . may not, in fact, do you much good. But, unless your doctor has forbidden it, it is unlikely to do much harm, so long as it is just 'a little' and you do not indulge yourself often. As the recipes in this book show, a healthy diet, which reduces the risk of developing cancer, can be a tasty diet, but, even so, eating completely healthy meals and snacks for seven days a week and 52 weeks a year can be a daunting prospect. So there is no point in worrying if you succumb to the urge to eat a packet of salty pretzels or a greasy hamburger – but only do it very occasionally, as a special treat. Try to make sure that at least 90 per cent of your diet is healthy.

DIET AND CANCER

Cancer is a condition in which normal cells change, or are changed by other chemicals (carcinogens), with the result that they multiply excessively, forming tumours. This may not, by itself, appear to be life-threatening. But when a cancer is malignant, rather than benign, it spreads and invades other tissues, attacking bone and blocking blood vessels and nerves until the body can no longer function.

Carcinogens, such as tobacco smoke, alcohol and environmental pollutants, can bring about these cellular changes. In the main, however, carcinogens in the diet are only very rarely a cause of cancer. The 15-year analysis of statistics relating to food intake and diet undertaken by the AICR has demonstrated that in a hugely significant proportion of cancer cases, the changes are the result of eating an unhealthy diet. Unfortunately, nobody knows for certain why this should be – perhaps ongoing research will provide the answer in the years ahead.

Here is a summary of the main findings of the AICR's study linking a reduction in the risks of specific cancers to dietary measures:

- **Lung cancer**: the most common cause of lung cancer is tobacco smoking, but a diet rich in vegetables and fruits may prevent between 20 and 33 per cent of cases in both smokers and non-smokers
- **Stomach cancer**: diets high in vegetables and fruits, and low in salt, together with the routine use of freezing and refrigeration of perishable foods may prevent between 66 and 75 per cent of cases
- **Breast cancer**: a diet rich in vegetables and fruit, an appropriate body weight and an avoidance of alcohol may prevent between 10 and 20 per cent of cases (more if this diet is adopted early in life)
- **Bowel cancer**: a diet high in fibre and vegetables and low in meat and alcohol may, together with regular physical exercise, prevent 66 to 75 per cent of cases
- **Mouth and throat cancer**: a diet high in vegetables and fruit and low in alcohol consumption may – in the absence of tobacco smoking – prevent between 30 and 50 per cent of cases
- **Liver cancer**: avoidance of alcohol (and of aflatoxins, found in a mould that grows on some types of nuts) may prevent between 33 and 66 per cent of cases.

The message seems fairly clear: if you smoke, stop now; moderate your alcohol intake; cut down on the amount of meat you eat; and emphasize vegetables and fruit in your diet. And it is particularly important that you take these steps if you have a family history of cancer, because genetic predisposition is a major risk factor for developing cancer.

Luckily, an anti-cancer diet is the same as the diet that doctors and nutritionists recommend for healthy living – and it is this same diet that can prevent numerous other conditions, such as high blood pressure, heart disease and diabetes. It relies on limiting your intake of certain carbohydrates and fats, and maximizing your intake of life-preserving vegetables and fruits and fibre and grains. In the following pages we will show you how to do just that – starting with a look at the chemicals, obtainable in a healthy diet, that actually prevent cancer from developing in the first place.

ANTIOXIDANTS, VITAMINS AND MINERALS

Many of our bodily structures can be damaged by the presence of what are known as 'free radicals' – technically speaking, these are atoms that have unpaired electrons. The most common free radical is radical oxygen, which can damage cells, causing them to develop cancerous changes, and increase the likelihood that cholesterol forms fatty plaques in arteries, leading to heart disease.

When this was realized, in the 1990s, nutritionists started to look at the antioxidants, which combat radical oxygen and so help prevent cancer and heart disease. These are known as 'phytochemicals', which literally means 'plant chemicals', and the most important antioxidants amongst them are vitamins C and E, beta-carotene (a precursor to vitamin A) and lycopene. Soon antioxidant supplements became increasingly popular, and today some 30 per cent of Americans take them. Unfortunately, they do not reduce the risks of cancer, heart disease or stroke, as a series of studies, and meta-studies (that is, studies of studies), have shown.

Nevertheless, it has been shown that a diet that is high in antioxidants is protective against cancer and heart disease. The answer to this conundrum is thought to be that in practice the effect of dietary antioxidants relies on the interaction between the antioxidants and other dietary ingredients: minerals, perhaps, or fibre. So it is important to eat a diet rich in antioxidants – that means richly coloured fruit and vegetables that contain chemicals called flavonoids, such as apricots, blueberries, bilberries, broccoli, carrots, mangoes, peppers and spinach, and, in particular, tomatoes (though these should be cooked to release maximum quantities of flavonoids). And, just to show that a healthy diet need not be without its luxuries, there are high levels of flavonoids in both dark chocolate and red wine – though both should be enjoyed in moderation.

Vitamins and minerals

Every one of our body's systems needs vitamins and minerals to function. Vitamins act as catalysts, initiating and controlling chemical reactions in the body, while minerals also play a vital part in body chemistry. Only small amounts of them are needed – they are known as micronutrients – and they must be obtained from our diet, because the body cannot manufacture them. If you follow the rules for healthy eating given in this book, and take a multivitamin supplement every day, as a precaution, you should absorb all the vitamins and minerals that your body requires. But sometimes the way that we treat and cook food reduces its content of micronutrients. Follow these rules to make sure that you can meet your body's requirements.

- Avoid processed foods, and canned foods in particular, because these can be low in vitamin content.
- Always use fresh or frozen fruit and vegetables, because vitamin levels decrease as these foods age. It is not generally realized that freezing preserves vitamin content, but chilling fruit and vegetables in a refrigerator before heating them can reduce levels of vitamins such as vitamin C and folic acid by up to 30 per cent. Remember that frozen vegetables – peas, especially – are often more vitamin-rich than fresh ones, because they are frozen immediately after being picked.
- Keep all foods away from heat, light and air, all of which reduce levels of vitamin C and the B vitamins. Store vegetables in airtight bags.
- Use the skin of fruits and vegetables wherever possible and avoid trimming them too much. Instead of peeling, wash or scrub them – most of the nutritional value of fruits and vegetables is contained in the skin or the area underneath it.
- Keep the water you have used to cook vegetables and use it as a base for stock or sauces – otherwise you will lose the valuable vitamins and minerals that have leached into the water.

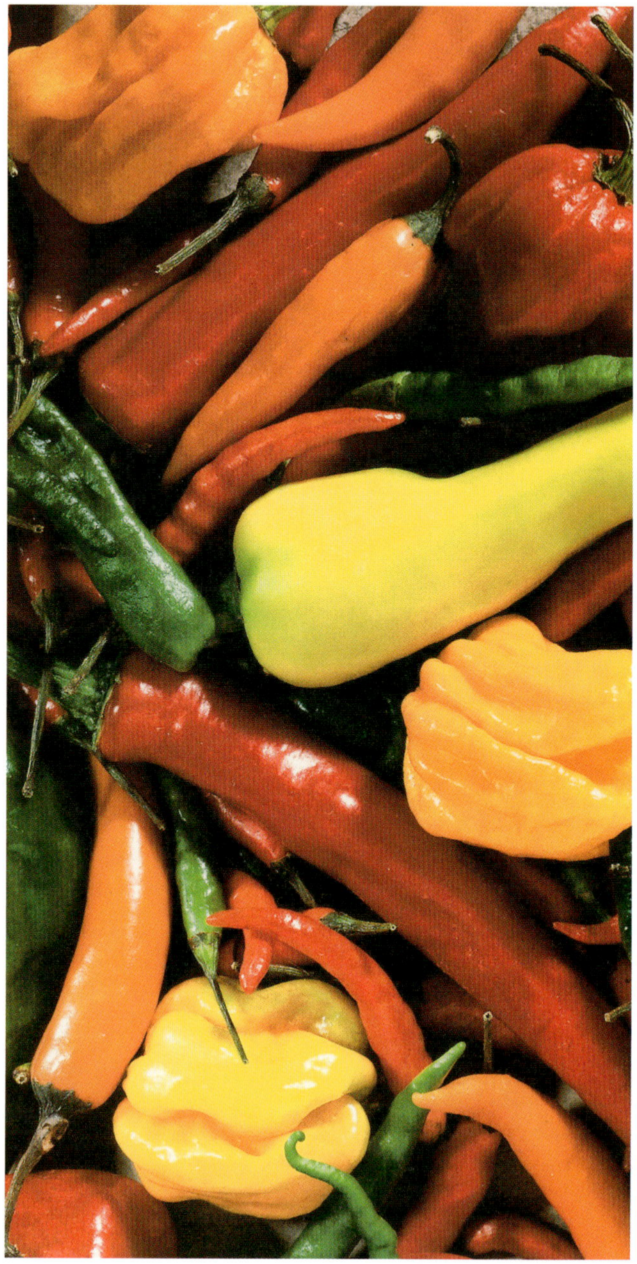

Richly coloured vegetables and fruit, such as these peppers, contain high levels of antioxidants which help prevent against cancer.

- Take a daily multivitamin supplement – it can be hard to obtain sufficient quantities of some vitamins, such as B12 and folic acid, from your diet; and fibre-rich foods contain chemicals called phytates, which can bind with some minerals and interfere with their absorption. But think of it as a nutritional safety net, rather than as a substitute for healthy eating.

VITAMIN- AND MINERAL-RICH FOODS

(NB Pre-menopausal women and women taking HRT should eat more of foods containing vitamins that are depleted by the female hormone oestrogen.)

Vitamin A (antioxidant)
Retinol: butter, cod liver oil and cheese
Beta-carotene: apricots, cantaloupe, carrots, kale, peach, peas, spinach and sweet potatoes

Vitamin B1
Beans, brown rice, milk, oatmeal, vegetables, whole grains and yeast (depleted by alcohol, caffeine, exposure to air and water, food additives and oestrogen)

Vitamin B2
Eggs, fish, meat, milk, vegetables, and whole grains (depleted by alcohol, caffeine, oestrogen and zinc)

Vitamin B3
Avocado, eggs, fish, meat, peanuts, prunes, seeds and whole grains (destroyed by canning and some sleeping pills; depleted by alcohol and oestrogen)

Vitamin B5
Bran, eggs, green vegetables, meat, whole grains and yeast (destroyed by canning)

Vitamin B6
Avocado, bananas, cabbage, cantaloupe, fish, milk, eggs, seeds and wheat bran (destroyed by alcohol, heat, oestrogen and processing techniques during production of commercial food)

Vitamin B folic acid
Apricots, avocados, beans, carrots, green vegetables, melons, oranges and whole wheat (destroyed by commercial food processing techniques, cooking and exposure to water and air, depleted by alcohol)

Vitamin B12
Dairy products, fish and meat (depleted by alcohol, exposure to sunlight and water, oestrogen and sleeping tablets)

Vitamin C (antioxidant)
Broccoli, cabbage, cauliflower, citrus fruits, green peppers, spinach, tomatoes, and potatoes (destroyed by boiling, exposure to air, and carbon dioxide and long storage; depleted by alcohol, aspirin, oestrogen, stress and tobacco)

Vitamin D
Cod liver oil, dairy products, and oily fish (depleted by lack of sunlight)

Vitamin E (antioxidant)
Almonds, broccoli, eggs, kale, oats, olive oil, peanuts, soybeans, seeds, spinach and wheat germ (destroyed by commercial food processing techniques, freezing, heat, oxygen, and chlorine; depleted by smoking and use of contraceptive pills)

Vitamin K
Broccoli, cod liver oil, eggs, green vegetables, live yoghurt, tomatoes and whole grains

Magnesium
Bitter chocolate, brown rice, nuts, soybeans and whole meal (depleted by caffeine and stress)

Zinc (antioxidant)
Eggs, meat, mushrooms, yeast and whole grains (inhibited by caffeine and smoking)

Potassium
Avocados, bananas, dried fruit, green vegetables, nuts and potatoes (lost in diarrhoea and sweat)

Selenium (antioxidant)
Broccoli, onions, tomatoes, tuna and wheat germ

TOO MUCH CAN BE DANGEROUS

Many people take high doses of vitamin supplements, without having taken medical advice. But doing so can be dangerous, because in many cases the effects of high doses are not known, and in some cases the effects have been confirmed to be dangerous. For example, it was once thought that very high doses of vitamin E might help prevent heart disease, but several studies have failed to show this and a recent study suggests that they may make heart failure more likely. And the list goes on: too much calcium can lead to lethargy, confusion and coma; excess vitamin B6 can cause a nerve disorder that leads to loss of feeling in the arms and legs; too much beta-carotene can increase the risk of contracting lung cancer in smokers; high doses of vitamin A can increase the risk of cardiovascular disease and can damage your liver; excessive doses of vitamin C can cause abdominal pain, nausea and diarrhoea; and so on.

The message is clear: do not take high-dose vitamin supplements unless they have been prescribed by your doctor – you can obtain all the antioxidants, vitamins and minerals you need by eating a healthy diet and taking a multivitamin supplement every day.

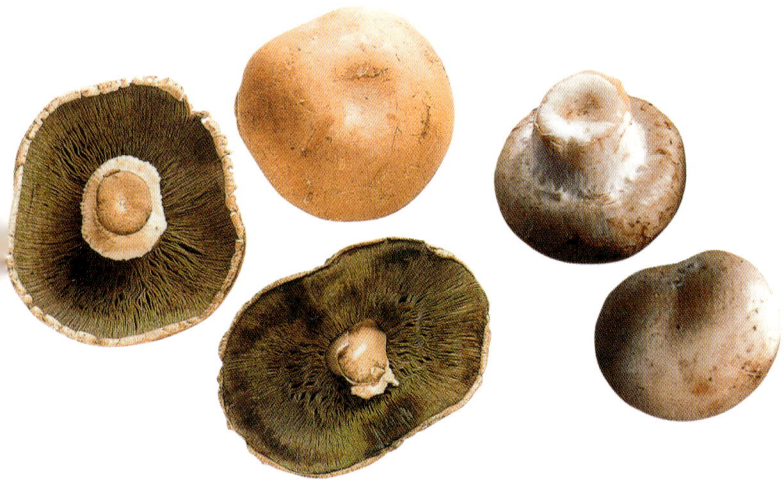

Mushrooms contain antioxidants, including zinc, but if you smoke these are inhibited.

CARBOHYDRATES

Carbohydrates are the body's primary source of fuel and are an essential part of a healthy diet. There are three types of carbohydrate: sugars, fibre and starch, and all of them are built from molecules of sugar. They used to be described as 'complex' or 'simple' carbohydrates, depending on whether they were simple forms of sugar or consisted of linked forms of sugar, and it was believed that simple carbohydrates should be avoided and complex ones preferred.

Today this categorization is now longer used. Instead, nutritionists classify carbohydrates according to their glycaemic index, or 'GI'. During the digestive process, carbohydrates are broken down into the simplest forms of sugar, and the glycaemic index measures how quickly this happens and so how fast levels of sugar in the blood rise – a high GI value means that the carbohydrate raises these levels very quickly.

The significance of this is that the pancreas starts to produce the hormone insulin in response to rising blood sugar levels, and this promotes the uptake of sugar by the body's cells and reduces sugar levels in the blood. If you continually eat foods with a high GI – and if you have a hereditary disposition to the problem or are overweight and inactive – the levels of both insulin and sugar in your blood remain high, and you develop what is known as insulin resistance (the body loses its sensitivity to insulin, so more and more is needed). This can not only lead to type 2 diabetes, but result in high blood pressure, low levels of 'good' cholesterol (see page 14) and the risk of heart disease.

There is some evidence that eating high GI carbohydrates may also be linked to an increased risk of colorectal, breast and pancreatic cancer, though the link has not been conclusively proved as yet. Until more is known, though, it would be sensible to choose a diet that emphasizes low and medium GI foods.

High or low?

In essence, whether a food has a high or low GI depends on how quickly its carbohydrates are converted to simple sugar during the digestive process. Foods that have not been processed – wholegrain foods – still contain their original fibre, which slows down the rate at which carbohydrates are converted to simple sugars and so also slows down the rate at which sugar enters the bloodstream; conversely, the carbohydrates in processed foods have already been partly broken down, meaning that their sugar enters the bloodstream relatively quickly.

However, the type of starch in the food is important, too: potatoes, for example, contain a starch that is broken down quickly during digestion. Other factors affecting the GI value are: ripeness – ripe fruit has a higher GI than unripe fruit; acidity – vinegar and lemon juice delay stomach emptying and so reduce the GI value; and the size of food particles – small particles are more easily absorbed and increase the GI value significantly.

Low GI foods include soy, beans, fruit, milk and grainy bread; medium ones include sugar, orange juice and oats; while high GI foods include potatoes, rice, and wholemeal and white bread. It might seem a daunting prospect to exist solely on low GI foods, but it is not necessary to do so. This is because eating a low GI food reduces the GI value of high GI foods when they are eaten at the same time – if, for example, you eat cornflakes (high GI) with milk (low GI) your blood sugar levels will not go up as quickly – what is known as the overall 'glycaemic load' (GL) is reduced. In essence, the equation reads 'high GI + low GI = medium GI' – so if you plan your menus carefully you can still eat some high GI foods.

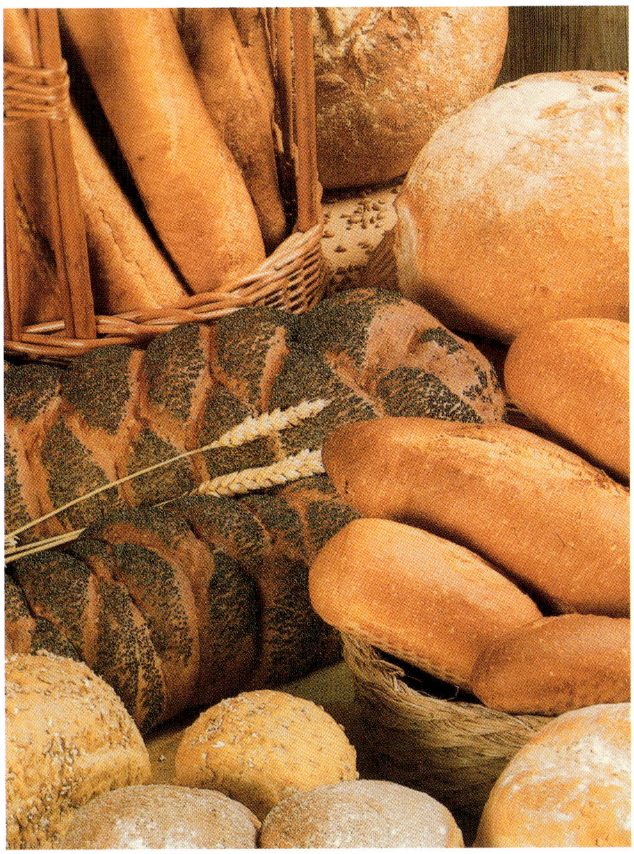

PLUSES AND A MINUS

Maximizing the amount of low GI foods in your diet and minimizing the amount of high GI ones has numerous benefits:

- the slow breakdown of low GI foods during digestion and the gradual release of their sugars into your bloodstream means that you will not feel the 'sugar let-down' that comes when quick-release sugars are used up; in turn this means that you will not need to have another 'sugar hit' as quickly, so you will eat less – which means that you will lose weight (about 450 to 900 g a week)
- the slow release of sugars into your bloodstream increases your physical endurance
- a low GI diet increases the body's sensitivity to insulin (see page 10), which reduces the risk of developing insulin resistance, and so diabetes and heart disease
- including a larger proportion of low GI foods means that you will reduce your intake of 'bad' saturated fats and trans fats (see page 14) and lessen the likelihood that you will develop heart disease
- there is some evidence that a low GI diet may help prevent some cancers
- so long as you choose low GI foods, you can snack between meals
- a low GI diet leads to increased levels of serotonin in the brain – and serotonin makes you feel good
- a low GI diet can easily be followed for life, unlike other fad diets.

But, in case low GI diet seems too good to be true, there is just one minus:

- healthy though they may be, even low GI foods contain calories, so if you eat too many of them you will not lose weight: you still have to control portion sizes.

White bread has a high glycaemic index value and therefore should be avoided, whereas wholewheat and granary are slightly better with a medium-high glycaemic index value.

CHECK THE LABEL

Food manufacturers are starting to note GI values on product labels, and the practice is likely to become more and more widespread. (In fact, the World Health Authority advises that GI values should be stated and that the values for 'complex carbohydrates' and sugars, which are used currently, are dropped.) But how do you interpret the figures?

The answer is that the maximum GI value, which is based on pure glucose, is 100, and that foods are said to have a low GI when the value is 55 or less; to be medium-GI when the value is between 56 and 69; and high-GI when the value is 70 or more.

Remember that, ideally, you should stick to low-GI foods; failing that, you should combine medium- and low-GI foods; and that if you ever eat high-GI foods you should combine them with low-GI ones.

FOODS TO CHOOSE

(Low glycaemic index carbohydrates)

Bran** and **porridge oats

Barley, buckwheat** and **bulgur wheat.

Some fruits – apples, citrus, berries, peaches, pears, plums and rhubarb

Pasta

Some vegetables – avocados, aubergine, beans (runner and green), broccoli, cabbage, cauliflower, carrots, celery, courgettes, cucumber, leeks, onions, lettuce, mushrooms, olives, peas, peppers, spinach and tomatoes

FOODS TO USE SPARINGLY

(Medium glycaemic index carbohydrates)

Pure wheat cereals.

Granary** and **wholemeal bread

Basmati** or **long-grained rice, wild rice and couscous

Corn – cornmeal, corn oil, sweetcorn

Some fruits – apricots, bananas, melon, dried fruit, pineapples, mangoes

Some vegetables – new potatoes, sweet potatoes, beetroot and artichokes

Honey

FOODS TO AVOID

(High glycaemic index carbohydrates)

Breakfast cereals – cornflakes and sugar-coated cereals

White bread, cakes, biscuits, bagels, buns, muffins, pancakes** and **doughnuts

White** and **brown rice

Some fruits – dates, prunes and watermelon

Gnocchi

Some vegetables – broad beans, potatoes (when mashed, baked, fried or roasted), parsnips and swede

Sugar – table, glucose, treacle and molasses

Tomato ketchup

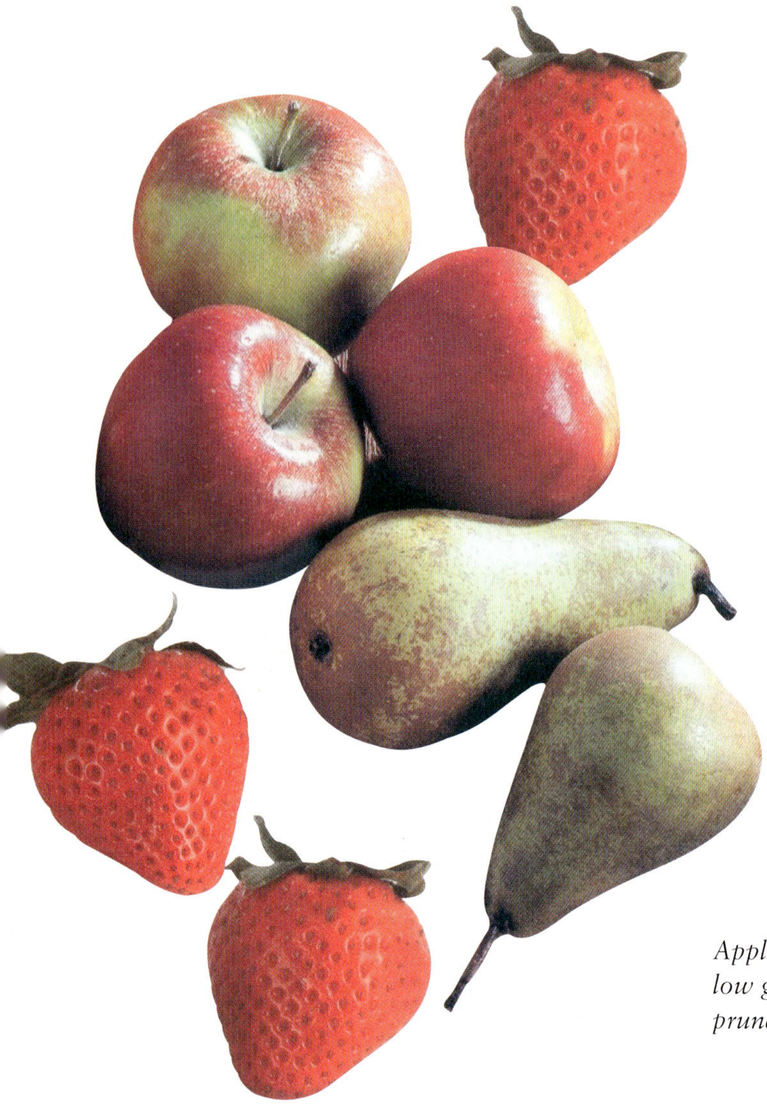

Apples, pears and strawberries contain carbohydrates with a low glycaemic index level; some fruits to avoid include dates, prunes and watermelon.

THE DANGERS OF BEING OVERWEIGHT

Being overweight brings with it the dangers of many health problems, including an increased risk of developing colonic and rectal cancer, but if you carry the extra pounds on your waist – in the classic 'beer belly' – you are far more at risk of heart disease or diabetes. In fact, men with waists of more than 101 cm (40 in) and women with waists of more than 89 cm (35 in) are at between double and quadruple the risk of developing them.

The reason is that fat that is stored around the stomach secretes hormones that play havoc with the production of insulin, the pancreatic hormone that controls blood sugar levels. As a result 'insulin resistance' develops, leading to diabetes, high blood pressure and high cholesterol levels. And the healthiest and most effective way to lose weight is to follow the low GI diet.

BLOOD PRESSURE

Most people know that high blood pressure puts the whole circulatory system at risk, causing a build-up of fatty plaques in the arteries and leading to heart disease or a stroke. What is less well known is that it is also a risk factor for certain cancers – in particular, for kidney cancer. But what is high blood pressure, and what causes it?

Pressure points

The phrase 'high blood pressure' means that the force that blood exerts on the walls of arteries as it flows through them is higher than is normal. Blood pressure values are expressed as two figures, representing millimetres of mercury in an old-fashioned blood pressure measuring device (a sphygmomanometer): 120/80, for example, is considered normal – the first figure is the systolic pressure, when the heart is pumping; the second is the diastolic pressure, when the heart is resting between beats. You are considered to have high blood pressure, and will be offered treatment for it, if your reading is 140/90 or higher. It is estimated that between 10 and 20 per cent of the population have high blood pressure, but many people do not know that they have it – there are often no symptoms, which is why it is sometimes known as 'the silent killer'.

Atherosclerosis is the condition in which plaques (atheromata) form on the inner walls of arteries. The plaques consist of dead cells, fibrous tissue and calcium, among other things, but primarily contain cholesterol. They can cause the arteries to harden, narrow and become less flexible (arteriosclerosis), or block them. If atherosclerosis blocks the coronary arteries, which supply the heart with blood, the result will be a heart attack. Sometimes, too, pieces of plaque can break off (thrombi) and be carried around the circulatory system to block other, smaller blood vessels – if these supply blood to the brain, the result could be a stroke.

The nature of the link between atherosclerosis and high blood pressure is complex. Each condition can cause the other one, but generally both develop as a result of lifestyle factors and the natural processes of ageing (some people also have an inherited predisposition to them). Smoking, drinking excessive amounts of alcohol, obesity, high stress levels, and the presence of other conditions, such as diabetes, play a major part in the development of both problems, but so, too, does your diet.

The culprits

The main dietary culprits when it comes to developing atherosclerosis and high blood pressure – and so some cancers – are saturated fats, trans fats, dietary cholesterol and salt. But some foods can actually prevent both problems. The trick is to know which foods to choose and which to avoid – and what follows will show you. Remember, too, that the more low GI foods you include in your diet, the less likely it is that you will eat 'bad' fats (see page 14).

FATS AND CHOLESTEROL

For many years, scientists believed that the cholesterol that you eat is the villain of the piece when it comes to heart disease. In fact, about 75 per cent of the cholesterol in your blood is manufactured by your liver, while only 25 per cent of it is in your diet. And the liver uses dietary fat to make cholesterol. When this was appreciated, the emphasis moved to eating a low-fat and low-cholesterol diet. But then it was discovered that it is not only the amount of fat in your diet that is important, but how much of which type of fat you eat – and there are three main types of fat: saturated fats, unsaturated fats and trans fats.

Saturated fats are found in meat, poultry, lard and whole-milk dairy products, such as cheese, milk, butter

KEEP CHECKING

There are often no symptoms if you have high blood pressure – which is why it is known as the silent killer. But it is important that you know what your blood pressure is, so that you can take steps to reduce it if it is too high. In Britain, it is recommended that everybody asks their family doctor to check their blood pressure every five years, and more frequently with age; in the US, the recommendation is that blood pressure should be checked every two years over the age of 20.

You can buy blood pressure monitors for home use, and a wide range of them is available on the internet. However, you should make sure to choose a model whose results have been validated by medical associations, because some models can give inaccurate results.

Blood levels

If your blood pressure is too high, a blood sample may be taken so that it can be tested for levels of cholesterol and tryglycerides (the form in which fats are transported in the blood). Depending on the result, you may be advised to adopt healthy eating measures and in some cases may be prescribed statin drugs, which control cholesterol levels.

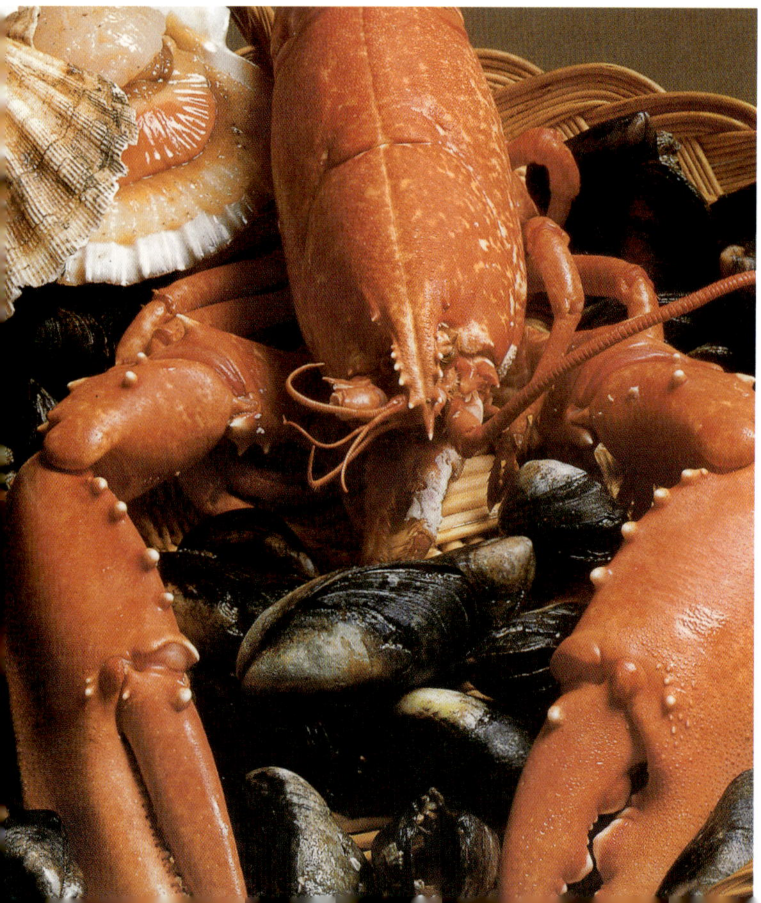

and cream, but high levels are also found in some vegetable oils, such as coconut and palm oil.

Unsaturated fats, which typically are liquid at room temperature, are found in plant and vegetable oils, such as olive, peanut, sesame, safflower, corn, sunflower, canola and soybean oil, and in avocados, oily fish (in the form of omega–3 fatty acid) and nuts and seeds.

Trans fats are man-made – a by-product of heating vegetable oils in the presence of hydrogen (which is why they are often referred to as 'hydrogenated vegetable oils' on product labels). They are found in commercially baked goods, such as biscuits, snack foods, processed foods and commercially prepared fried foods, such as crisps. Some margarines also contain high levels of trans fats, especially brands that are 'stick' margarines – spreadable ones have less high levels as they are less hydrogenated (hydrogenation makes the fat hard at room temperature).

Where cholesterol comes in

Your body needs cholesterol to function correctly – it is involved in the production of hormones, the body's chemical messengers, as well as bile and vitamin D, and is found in every part of the body. For this reason, it is manufactured in the liver – and the liver uses fats to make it. If you eat too much saturated fat, the liver produces too much cholesterol. And, unfortunately, cholesterol is a soft, waxy substance that can stick to the lining of blood vessels and obstruct them if there are high levels of it in the blood.

As we have seen, liver-produced cholesterol, and so the cholesterol that is ultimately the result of fat consumption, accounts for around 75 per cent of the cholesterol found in your blood. The remaining 25 per cent comes from the cholesterol you eat. Dietary cholesterol is found in eggs, dairy products, meat, poultry, fish and shellfish, but the highest levels are found in egg yolks, meats such as liver and kidneys and shellfish. Vegetables, fruits, nuts, grains and cereals contain no cholesterol.

'Good' and 'bad' cholesterol

Cholesterol is carried around the body by chemicals called lipoproteins. There are two types: low-density lipoprotein (LDL) and high-density lipoprotein (HDL).

Suprisingly, shellfish contain high cholestorol levels along with egg yolks, kidneys and liver, and therefore should be eaten in moderation.

If there is too much of the cholesterol carried by LDL, known as 'bad' cholesterol, plaque builds up on arterial walls. But HDL carries cholesterol away from the arteries to the liver, which breaks it down so that it can be excreted from the body; for this reason, HDL cholesterol is said to be 'good' cholesterol. It is now known that saturated fats, and, in particular, trans fats, increase the blood levels of harmful LDL cholesterol and lower levels of beneficial HDL cholesterol, while unsaturated fats have the opposite effect.

To sum up, then, a healthy diet, which helps prevent heart disease and some cancers, is one that has low levels of saturated and trans fats, and high levels of unsaturated fats.

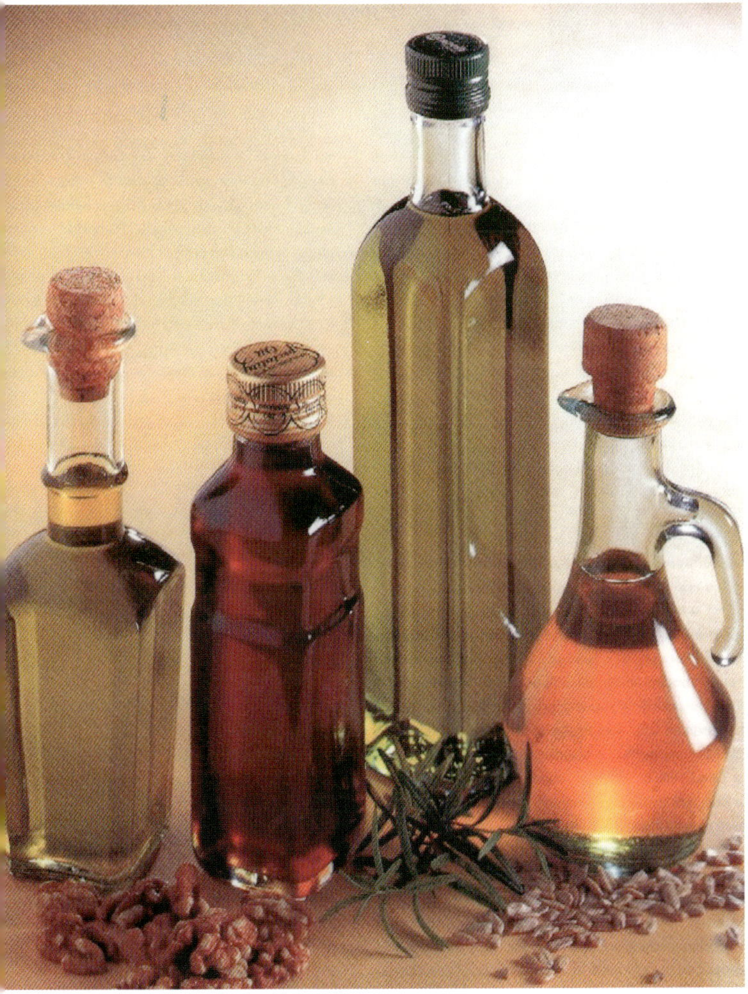

These oils, olive, safflower, walnut and sesame, contain unsaturated fats, which increase the levels of beneficial HDL cholesterol while lowering the blood levels of harmful LDL cholesterol.

FOODS TO CHOOSE

(Containing unsaturated fat)

Vegetable oils – pure olive, peanut, walnut, sesame, corn, soybean, sunflower and safflower oils

Avocados

Oily fish – salmon, mackerel, tuna, herrings and so on

Nuts** and **seeds

Spreadable, unsaturated margarine

FOODS TO USE SPARINGLY

(Containing saturated fat)

Whole-fat milk *(skimmed milk is preferable)*

Butter, cream, cheese, full-fat yoghurt *(low-fat is preferable) and* ***ice cream***

Meat – beef, lamb and pork

Poultry – battery-farmed chicken (free-range is preferable), goose, duck and turkey (wild game, such as rabbit, wild duck and venison, is better)

Lard

Eggs *(especially ones from battery-farmed chickens)*

Coconut oil *and* ***palm oil***

FOODS TO AVOID

(Containing trans fats)

Ready-made commercial foods – cakes, biscuits, and snack foods

Processed foods – sausages, pâté, scotch eggs, pies and so on

Commercially prepared fried foods – crisps, battered fish and chips

Hard margarine

FOODS TO USE SPARINGLY

(Rich in dietary cholesterol)

Organ meats – liver and kidneys

Eggs *(especially ones from battery-farmed chickens)*

Shellfish

Red meat

SALT

The more salt you eat, the more your body retains fluid, and the more fluid there is, the harder your heart has to work to pump blood around your body. And the result of this increase in the heart's work rate is high blood pressure and the risk, over time, of developing heart failure. High levels of salt in your diet are also linked to the incidence of certain cancers – in particular to stomach cancer.

Doctors recommend that our daily intake of salt should be less than 6 grams – about a teaspoonful. Even less salt than this is recommended for those who already have heart problems. The level is lower for children, too: up to 6 months old, it is less than 1 gram; between 7 and 12 months it is 1 gram; between 1 and 3 years it is 2 grams; between 4 and 6 it is 3 grams; and between 7 and 10 years it is 5 grams. Worryingly, one small can of spaghetti hoops served on a piece of toast made from white, supermarket bread contains around 0.9 grams – half of a toddler's recommended daily intake.

Hidden salt

The 6 gram target sounds an easy enough one to achieve, but in fact it is a very tall order. The reason is that this target refers to our total salt intake, not just to the salt that we add to our food, and there is a considerable amount of salt hidden in the foods many of us eat. Processed foods are mainly to blame – in fact, researchers estimate that around 75 per cent of our salt intake comes from them.

It is obvious that some foods contain high salt levels: salted nuts, crisps, olives and anchovies, for example, all taste, and are, salty. But bacon, cheese, pickles, stock cubes, sausages and smoked meat and fish contain salt, too. And some brands of biscuits, pizzas, 'ready meals', soups and breakfast cereals are also surprisingly high in salt.

The only way to check which processed foods are high in salt is to read product labels carefully. It is easy to come unstuck when you do this, however, because some labels do not refer to the product's salt content but to its sodium content (salt is made up of sodium and chloride). The two values are not the same – in fact, you have to multiply the sodium value by 2.5 to obtain the real salt content.

Reducing your salt intake

If you cut down on salt, your blood pressure will fall within weeks, even if it was not too high in the first place. And that means that your risk of developing heart disease, having a stroke or developing certain cancers will also fall.

Many people think that their food will lack taste if they cut down on salt, but this is a myth. You may find that your diet is a little bland for the first week or so, but your taste buds soon adapt. Adopt these salt reduction strategies and you will find the process much more easy.

- **Avoid** processed foods
- **Check** the salt levels of all commercially prepared foods, including everyday products such as bread
- **Throw** away your salt shaker
- **Make** your own salt-free stocks and sauces

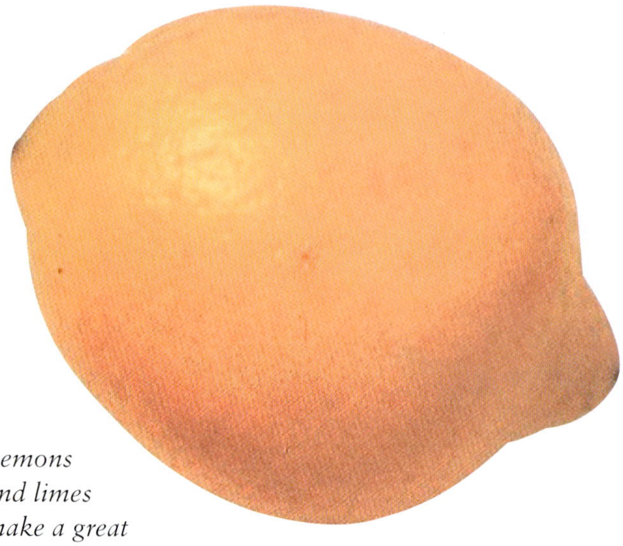

Lemons and limes make a great alternative to salad cream and mayonnaise, and they make great marinades for meats. Their sour flavour can also be used as a salt substitute.

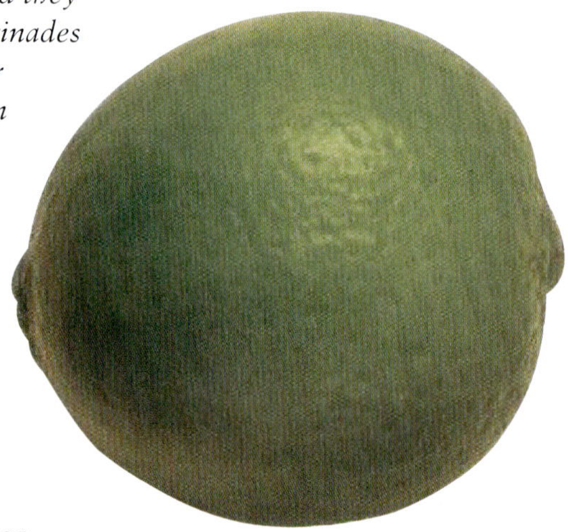

CALCULATE YOUR SALT INTAKE

If you must eat processed foods – and it can be hard not to – try to make sure that you stay within the recommended daily intake of 6 grams of salt. Read a product's label to find the number of grams of salt in 100 grams of the contents. If the quantity of sodium is given, multiply by 2.5 to calculate the actual salt content. (If the value is given in milligrams, or 'mg', divide by 1,000 to convert it to grams.)

Then look for the total weight of the contents, or estimate the proportion of them that you intend to use. Divide the weight that you will use by 100, then multiply by the number of grams of salt in each 100 grams and you will discover how much salt you will eat. The results can be surprising: one small (200 g) can of baked beans can contain as much as 1.7 grams of salt – just under a third of your total recommended intake; one slice of white, refined bread contains 0.61 grams of salt – so just the bread making up a lunchtime sandwich could well account for just under a fifth of your total recommended daily intake.

FOODS TO AVOID

All types of salt – table, rock, sea and garlic
Obviously salty foods – anchovies, salted nuts and ready-salted crisps

FOODS TO USE SPARINGLY

(High in salt)
Commercially made foods – biscuits, supermarket bread, cheese crackers and crisps
Ready-made meals – including pasta, pizzas, curries and Asian cuisine
Tinned foods – baked beans, spaghetti, meats and vegetables
Preserved and smoked foods – bacon, ham, pickles, spiced sausage, stock cubes and sauces

As well as reducing the amount of salt you eat, you should also cut down your red meat intake and get your protein from foods such as beans and pulses.

- **Use** alternative seasonings, such as lemon juice, herbs and vinegar
- **Eat** fresh fruit (bananas and avocados in particular) and vegetables: the potassium they contain helps counter the effect of dietary salt
- **Do** not switch to sea salt, rock salt or garlic salt – they are not different to normal salt
- **Ask** your doctor whether salt substitutes are suitable for you.

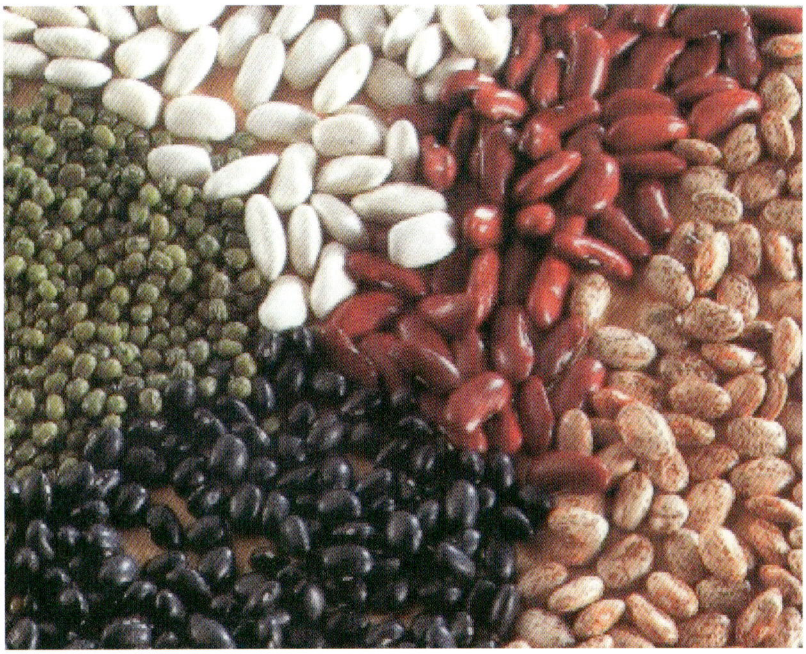

SALT SUBSTITUTES

Some people find that their food tastes a little bland when they switch to a low-salt diet, and even though their taste buds will adapt within a few weeks some people find that they need a little help to make the change. A number of salt substitutes are on the market, but these contain part sodium and part potassium and in certain circumstances it is possible to overload your body with potassium – consult your doctor before using a commercial salt substitute.

Make your own

This recipe for a salt substitute relies on the principle that a sour flavour is a good substitute for a salty one. It uses the grapefruit peel (or lemon or orange peel, for a weaker taste) and citric acid crystal. Also known as 'sour salt' and 'lemon salt', these can be found in the baking section of supermarkets or in delicatessens.

Ingredients

- the peel of 1 grapefruit
- 1 tbsp ground allspice
- 1/2 tbsp citric acid crystals

Makes 3 tablespoons

Method

1 Peel the grapefruit as thinly as possible, then scrape away all the white parts. Dry the peel overnight near a source of heat.

2 Grind the dried peel in a coffee grinder or spice grinder, then combine it with the other ingredients. Put the mixture into a well-sealed bottle and shake well to mix. Store in a dry place.

Variations

Add a tablespoon of freshly ground black pepper to the mixture to make it into citrus pepper, an ideal seasoning for meat.

PROTEIN

Protein, made up from chemicals called amino acids, makes up the building blocks of all our body's tissues except stored fat. You need to eat a certain amount of protein every day – a minimum of one gram for every kilogram of body weight – to prevent the body from starting to break down tissue. And you need more than that if you want to build up healthy muscles and robust bones.

It is easy to get enough protein in your diet in Western industrialized societies, though hard to do so in developing countries. But the quantity of protein you eat is not the whole story. What is important is that you eat a variety of amino acids, which means protein from a variety of sources. This does not mean that it is essential to eat steaks, for example, because you can obtain a full range of proteins from vegetable and fruit sources, if you are a vegetarian. Variety is the watchword.

FOODS TO CHOOSE

('Good' protein – lower in saturated fats)

Vegetables – beans, brown rice, lentils, millet and pulses

Soybeans

Nuts – brazil, peanuts and pinenuts

Seeds – sesame

Free-range chicken and turkey *(but remove the skin)*

Locally sourced lean cuts of non-intensively reared meats – beef, lamb, pork and veal

Free-range chicken eggs *(but not duck or goose eggs)*

FIBRE

Our bodies cannot digest some of the food that we eat, and it is this indigestible material that is known as dietary fibre. Most people know that a diet high in fibre is good for your bowel function and can protect against disorders of the intestines, such as cancer of the colon, but it is less well known that fibre can also lower the levels of cholesterol in your blood – which will lower your blood pressure and reduce your risk of developing other cancers, too.

There are two types of fibre: insoluble and soluble (the latter is so-called because it forms a gel when mixed with liquid). Insoluble fibre plays the main part

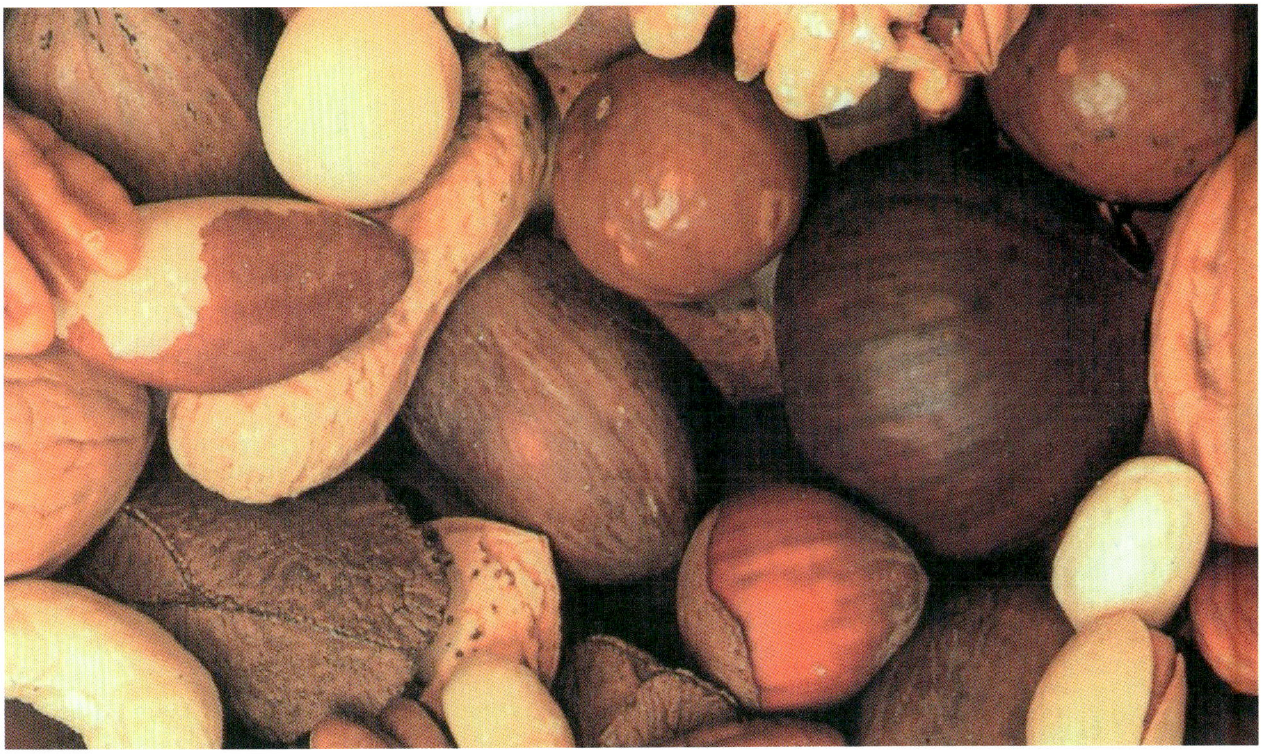

Nuts are high in soluble fibre, and also high in vitamins and minerals such as potassium and magnesium. Vitamin B3 can be found in peanuts; vitamin E in peanuts and almonds; and selenium in Brazil nuts.

in promoting bowel function, and high levels of it are found in foods such as wholemeal bread, wheat cereals, rice, barley, grains, cabbage, carrots, and so on. But it is soluble fibre that reduces blood cholesterol – though it is not clear how it does this. It is found in oats, oat bran, oatmeal, peas, beans, barley and fruits, and, conveniently, foods containing soluble fibre have a low GI rating.

Five a day

So it makes sense to increase your intake of foods rich in fibre, and especially of those rich in soluble fibre – generally, it is recommended that you should eat five portions of fibre-rich fruit and vegetables a day. And, of course, foods such as these are low in saturated fats and cholesterol. Make sure that you read labels carefully, though, because some commercial products that claim to be rich in fibre in fact contain very little of it.

FOODS TO CHOOSE

(High in soluble fibre)

Oatmeal *and* ***oat bran***

Lentils, beans *and* ***peas***

Apples, bananas, blueberries, oranges, pears *and* ***strawberries***

Sweetcorn, spinach, spring greens, *and* ***broccoli***

Nuts – almonds, brazil, hazel, peanuts, pecan, pistachio and walnuts

Seeds – sesame, sunflower and pumpkin

FOODS TO USE

(High in insoluble fibre)

Whole grains – bran, wheat, couscous, brown rice, bulgur and barley

Wholemeal *and* ***granary bread***

Wholemeal pasta

Wholemeal flour

Wholegrain breakfast cereals

Fruit – both fresh and dried

All vegetables – but especially brussel sprouts, carrots, cabbage, okra, parsnips, sweetcorn, courgettes, cucumber, celery, tomatoes and unpeeled potatoes

STRIKING A BALANCE

It is easy to decide which foods you should eat, but more difficult to decide how often to eat them. It is also hard to strike a nutritional balance between foods so that you obtain all the nutrients that your body demands in the correct quantities, yet protect your heart and arteries at the same time. And you will have noticed already from the tables in this book that certain foods are 'good' in the sense that they contain substantial quantities of a desirable ingredient, but 'not so good' in that they contain less desirable ingredients. So how do you do it?

The healthy eating pyramid shown on the opposite page indicates how often you should eat the different food groups. For instance, while foods such as cheese and other dairy products are important as part of a balanced diet, you should try to use these only sparingly because of the high levels of saturated fat they contain.

A diet high in antioxidants can help reduce the amount of cancer-causing substances in the body. All the recipes in this book are specifically designed to give you high levels of antioxidants, and they show that a healthy diet can be full of variety and flavour.

EXPLAINING THE SYMBOLS

SOLUBLE FIBRE

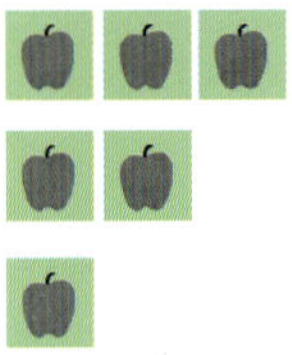

HIGH

MEDIUM

LOW

PROTEIN

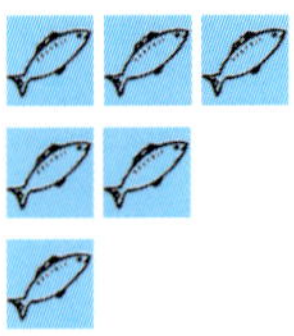

HIGH

MEDIUM

LOW

ANTIOXIDANT

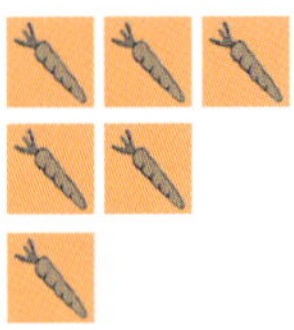

HIGH

MEDIUM

LOW

SATURATED FAT

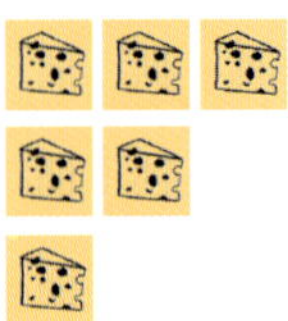

HIGH

MEDIUM

LOW

UNSATURATED FAT

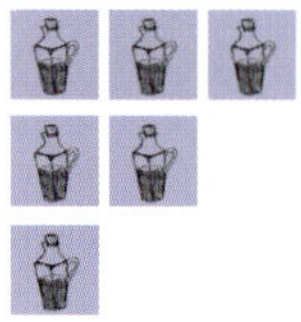

HIGH

MEDIUM

LOW

CHOLESTEROL

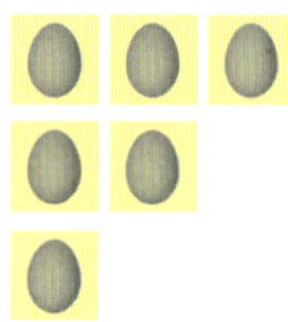

HIGH

MEDIUM

LOW

GLYCAEMIC INDEX

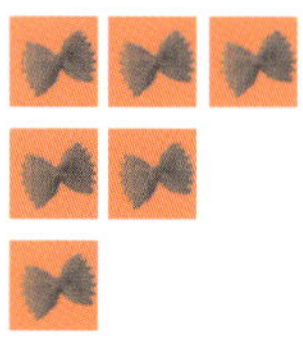

HIGH

MEDIUM

LOW

INSOLUBLE FIBRE

HIGH

MEDIUM

LOW

HEALTHY EATING PYRAMID

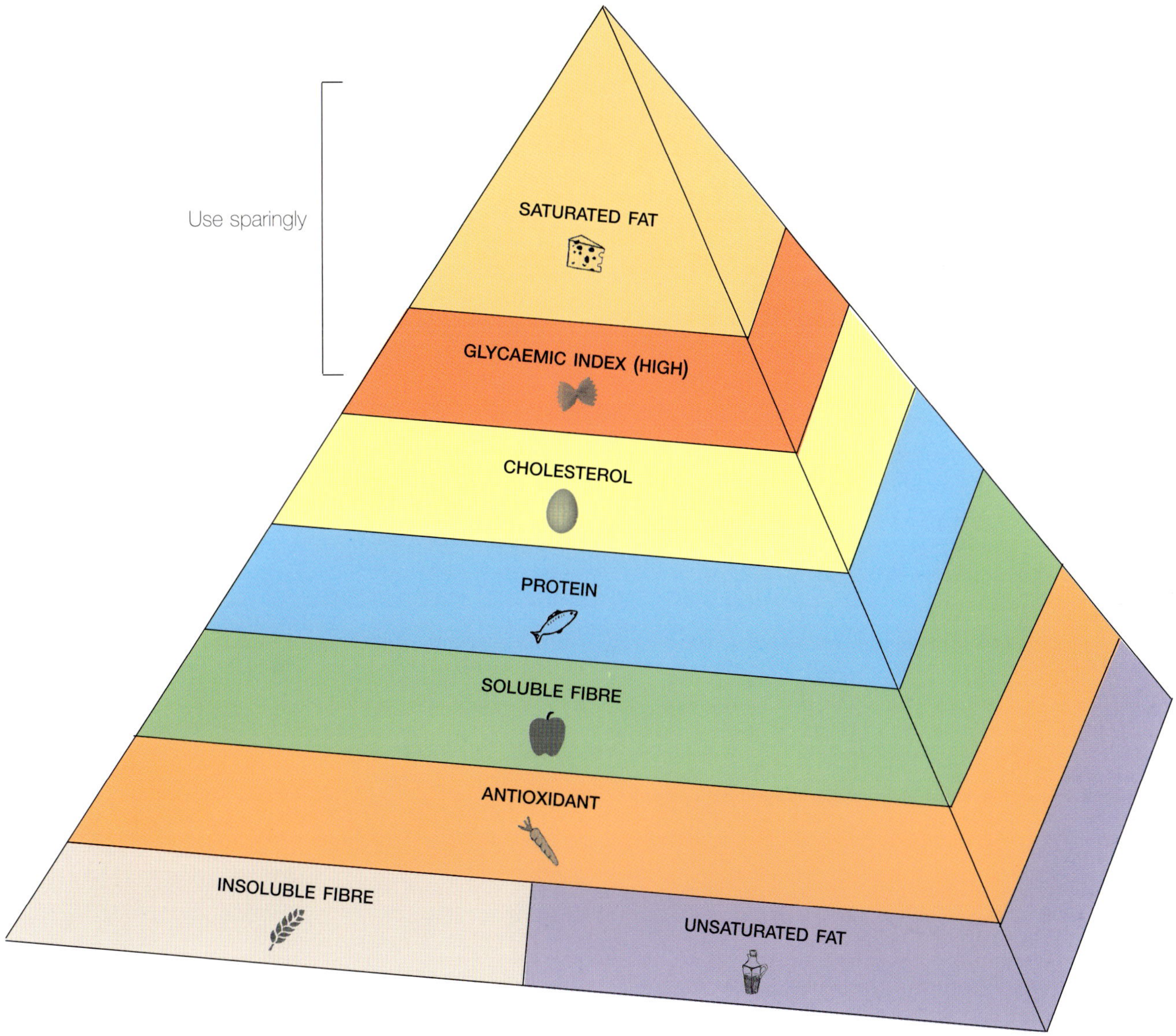

Saturated Fat: Red meat, goose, duck, cheese, butter, cream, full-fat yoghurt

Glycaemic Index (HIGH): Rice, white bread, potatoes, desserts, broad beans, prunes, watermelon and pasta

Cholesterol: Eggs, butter, cream, cheese, shellfish, pork, lamb, beef (0–1 times daily)

Protein: Fish, shellfish, free-range chicken, rabbit, wild game, low-fat dairy (1–2 times daily)

Soluble Fibre: Oats, barley, peas, beans, fruits (e.g. apples, oranges, bananas) nuts (2–3 times daily)

Antioxidant: Spinach, broccoli, garlic, onions, red and orange vegetables and fruit, berries (at most meals)

Insoluble Fibre: Wheat bran, wholemeal flour, wild rice, grains, cabbage, cauliflower, fruit skins (at most meals)

Unsaturated Fat: Olive oil, soya beans, avocado, peanuts, salmon, mackerel, tuna, sardines (1–2 times daily)

HOW TO COOK HEALTHILY

There is little point in choosing healthy ingredients and recipes if you cook them in a way that is in itself unhealthy. It is important to choose cooking methods that not only help reduce cholesterol and saturated fats and keep the calorie count low, but maximize the nutritional value of each dish. These techniques are effective, but may require a little practice:

- Baking – good for vegetables, fruit, poultry and lean meat, as well as for puddings; you may need a little extra liquid
- Braising or stewing – brown first, on top of the stove, then cook in a small quantity of liquid; if you leave the dish in a refrigerator you can remove the chilled fat and then reheat it
- Grilling – on a rack, so that fat can drain away, and not in a direct flame
- Microwaving – place the food between two paper towels to drain fat away while it cooks
- Poaching – in a covered pan of the correct size, so that you use the minimum liquid
- Roasting – on a rack so that the food does not sit in fat; baste with fat-free liquids, such as wine or lemon juice
- Sautéing – use a high heat and a small amount of non-stick cooking spray, or just cook without spray if you have a good-quality non-stick pan
- Steaming – in a perforated basket over simmering water; add seasoning to the water for extra flavour
- Stir-frying – in a wok, using a small amount of non-stick cooking spray or a tiny amount of olive oil.

You can also increase flavour, reduce fat and salt content and make the most of your ingredients' nutritional value if you

Remember to:

- Avoid cooking methods that char food, such as barbecuing or grilling over a direct flame – charring produces carcinogens
- Check labels for common ingredients, such as soy sauce, baking soda and monosodium glutamate – these all contain high levels of sodium and should be used very sparingly, if at all
- Make your own stock rather than using pre-prepared cubes, which can be high in salt
- Steam vegetables, for preference, in order to maximize both their flavour and nutritional value
- Cook lightly to preserve vitamin content (but cook meats and other foods that may harbour disease-producing organisms thoroughly)
- Choose extra virgin olive oil and vinegar rather than salted, pre-prepared salad dressings
- Wash canned vegetables before use – by doing so you can substantially reduce their salt content
- Use only one egg yolk when making scrambled eggs or omelettes, but mix in two or three extra egg whites
- Trim as much fat as you can from meat before you cook it and remove the skin from poultry
- Choose lean, low-fat meats, such as game (but, again, remember to remove the skin) and venison
- Drain oil from canned fish and rinse the fish in water before you use it
- Use herbs, wine and freshly ground pepper to enhance flavours; remember that a dash of vinegar or lemon juice will not only enhance flavour but reduce the GI rating of other ingredients.

Garlic can be used to flavour your cooking, rather than using salt. There is also evidence to suggest that it may be good for the heart.

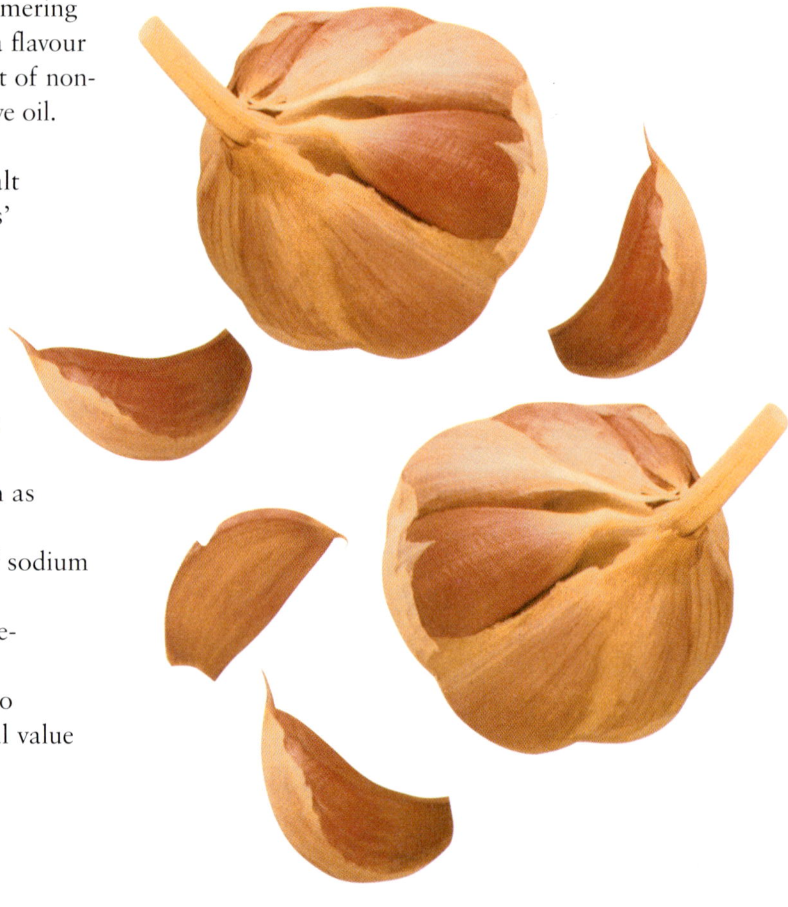

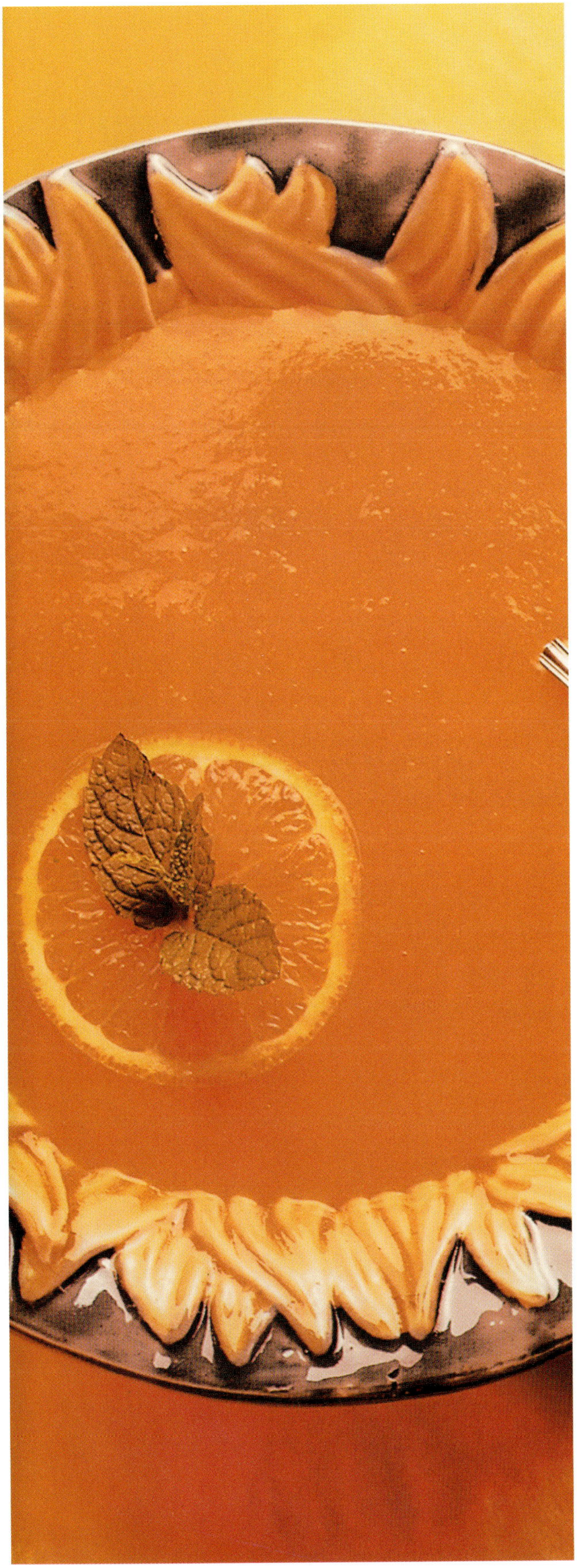

MAKE YOUR OWN STOCK

Many stock cubes contain high levels of salt and low levels of nutrients. But nothing could be more simple than making your own stock, and if you make it in large batches you can freeze it for later use. You can use your stock as the basis for a delicious soup – serve it with a wholegrain roll – or as the basis of a nourishing stew or a piquant sauce.

VEGETABLE STOCK

Ingredients

3 large carrots, scrubbed but not peeled, coarsely chopped
1 turnip, coarsely chopped
2 onions, coarsely chopped
2 leeks, coarsely chopped
4 ribs of celery, including tops, coarsely chopped
coarsely chopped trimmings from cauliflower, spinach, broccoli or any other vegetables, so long as they are fresh and clean. Always use fresh vegetables.
1 cup any dried beans, having been soaked overnight, if necessary; or use rice or barley
2 Tbsp olive oil
1 bouquet garni, which includes 3 sprigs parsley, 1 sprig thyme and 1 bay leaf
1 Tbsp peppercorns
Approx 3.5 litres cold water for 900 g vegetables

Method

Warm the olive oil in a stockpot, add the vegetables and simmer, stirring continuously for 15 minutes until they start to colour slightly. Then add the water and the other ingredients and bring to simmering point. Simmer for at least 2 hours, adding more water if necessary. Then strain through cheesecloth or use a non-metallic colander. Use or freeze, as required.

When making soup, always try to us fresh vegetables rather than canned or frozen ones.

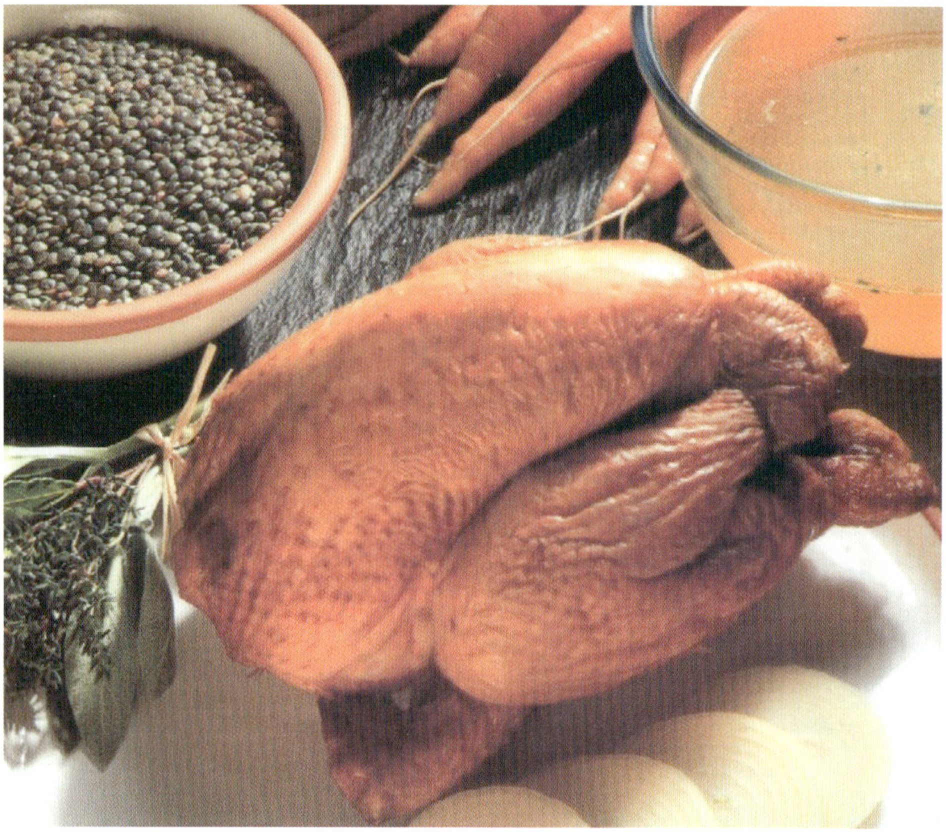

Use the stocks for the basis of soups and stews. Soups are easy to make and are great as starters or main courses. Soups made using fresh vegetables are not only healthier, but also much tastier.

CHICKEN STOCK

Ingredients

The bones of a chicken, and, if available, a ham bone or a veal knuckle (ask your butcher for one)
2 leeks, coarsely chopped
2 large carrots, scrubbed but not peeled, coarsely chopped
3 large onions, coarsely chopped
2 ribs of celery, tops included, coarsely chopped
6 sprigs of parsley, coarsely chopped
1 large clove garlic
2 cloves
1 Tbsp peppercorns
Lemon rind from half a lemon

Method

Place the bones in a stockpot and cover with cold water. Bring to simmering point – do not allow to boil. Simmer for at least an hour, then add all other ingredients and more cold water to cover, if necessary. Return to simmering point and simmer for another 2 hours. Then strain through cheese-cloth or use a non-metallic colander. Refrigerate, and when stock has set remove any fat from the top. Use or freeze, as required.

FISH STOCK

Ingredients

900 g fish bones, heads (with gills removed) and tails (sole or plaice are tastiest, but any other white, non-oily fish will do)
1 large onion, coarsely chopped
2 shallots, coarsely chopped
2 ribs of celery, tops included, coarsely chopped
2 large carrots, scrubbed but not peeled, coarsely chopped
2 bay leaves
2 cloves
6 sprigs of parsley, coarsely chopped
1 Tbsp peppercorns
Lemon rind from half a lemon
Cold water to cover

Method

Place everything in a stockpot and bring to simmering point – do not allow to boil. Simmer for 20–30 minutes, but no longer or the stock will become bitter. Strain through cheese-cloth or use a non-metallic colander. Reduce the strained stock by boiling, if required. Use or freeze as required.

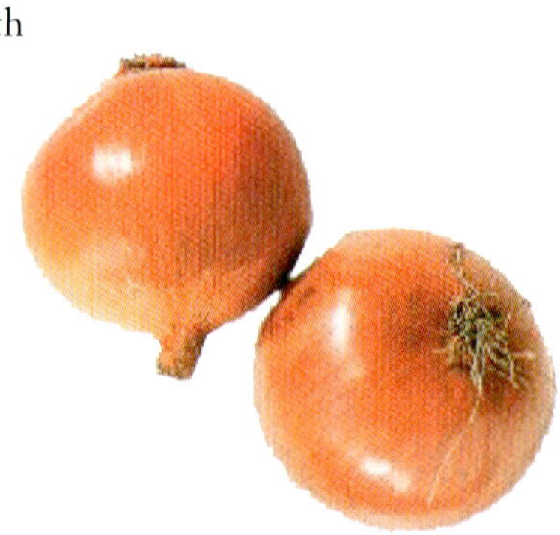

A HEALTHY LIFESTYLE

Eating a healthy diet is only one part of a healthy lifestyle. To reduce the risk of developing cancer and high blood pressure, to lower cholesterol levels, promote cardiovascular health and improve the quality of your life, you should also:

- **Give up smoking** – if you smoke, you are massively increasing the risk that you will develop lung, mouth, or throat cancer, and more than doubling the risk of having a heart attack, and you are more likely not to survive a heart attack

- **Manage stress** – use relaxation techniques and anger-management methods to cope with stress and keep your blood pressure low

- **Lose weight** – if you are overweight, you are more at risk of developing certain cancers and between two and six times more likely to develop high blood pressure

- **Cut down on alcohol** – there's evidence to suggest that two units of alcohol, and especially of red wine, can reduce blood pressure, but more than this can increase the risk of certain cancers and actually raise blood pressure

- **Lead an active life** – even small amounts of physical activity, for example walking or gardening, can increase the number of calories that you burn and so help lose weight, as well as reducing the risk of developing cancers and heart disease.

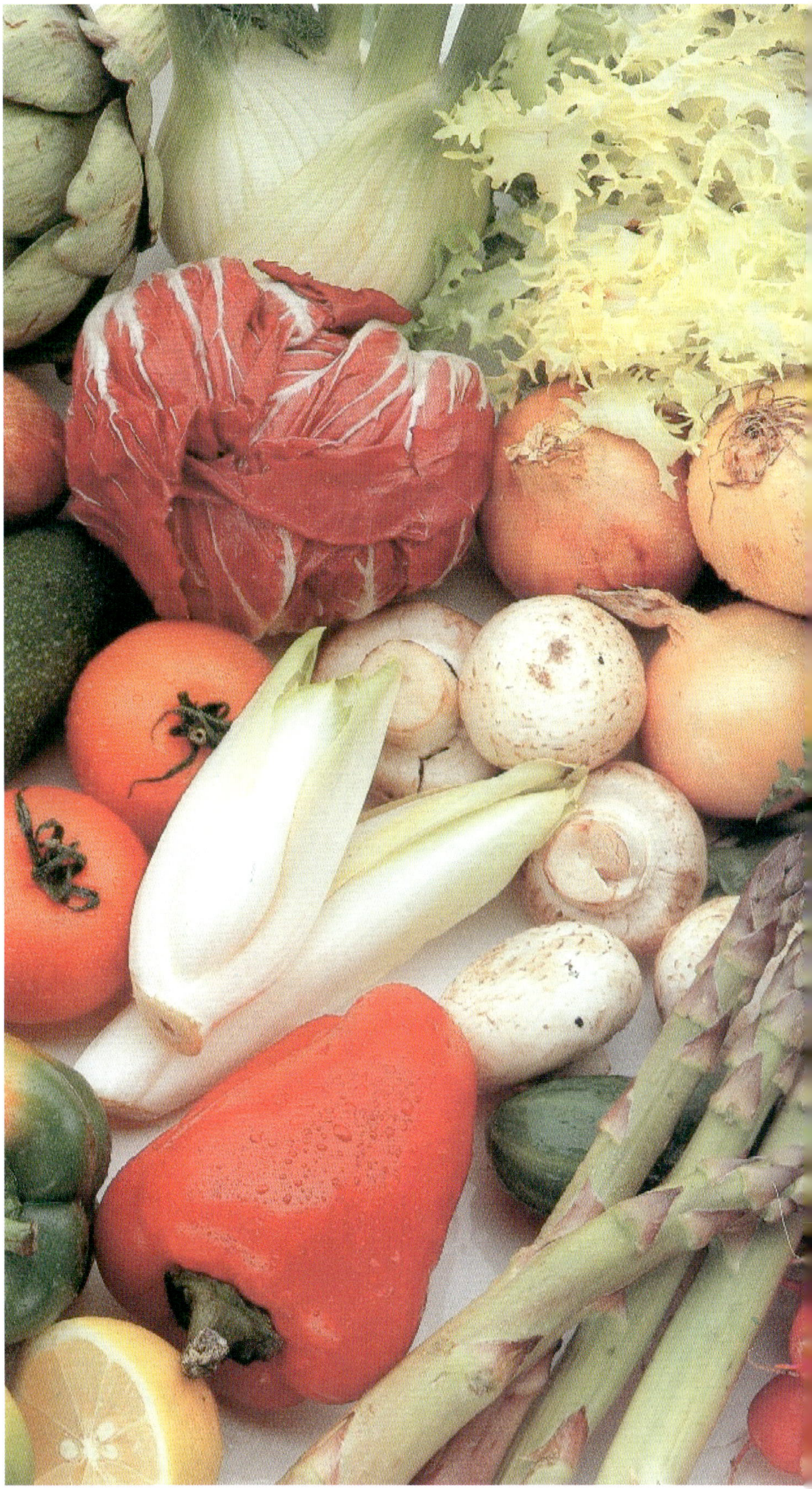

Fruit and vegetables are an essential part of a healthy diet. But for a healthy diet to be truly effective it is important that you make other changes to your lifestyle, including exercising, reducing your intake of alcohol and giving up smoking.

TABLES

These tables give the nutritional values for the main ingredients used in the recipes that follow. To eat healthily and minimize your risk of developing cancer, the major part of your diet should consist of foods with a high fibre content, a low fat content, moderate protein levels, a low or medium glycaemic index and plenty of antioxidants. Use the Healthy Eating Pyramid on page 21 as a guide to proportions.

Remember that carrying excess weight is a major risk for developing ill health, and watch your calorie intake, too. Doctors recommend that men with a sedentary lifestyle – that of an office worker, say – should eat 2,700 calories a day, while women should eat 2,000. In order to lose weight gradually, at the rate of half a kg a week, you need to reduce this figure by 500 calories.

Food	Quantity	Glycaemic index	Fat	Protein	Fibre	Calories
Meat and Dairy						
Cheese, feta	20 g	M	6	4	0	80
Cheese, reduced fat	20 g	M	4.5	7	0	70
Chicken, skinless	100 g	L	5	30	0	150
Crème fraîche, low fat	100 g	M	17.5	3	0	800
Egg	1 medium	M	5.5	6	0	80
Lean beef, lamb, pork	100 g	M	7	30	0	190
Milk, low fat	250 ml	L	2.5	8	0	102
Rabbit	100 g	L	4.5	30	0	160
Wild fowl	100 g	L	6	30	0	155
Yoghurt	100 g	L	0	5	0	40
Fish						
Herring, salmon	100 g	L	11	20	0	180
Mackerel	100 g	L	18	25	0	220
Sardine	100 g	L	2	15	0	65
Shellfish	100 g	L	1	15	0	105
Trout	100 g	L	6	20	0	155
Tuna	100 g	L	3	20	0	120
White fish	100 g	L	2	20	0	90

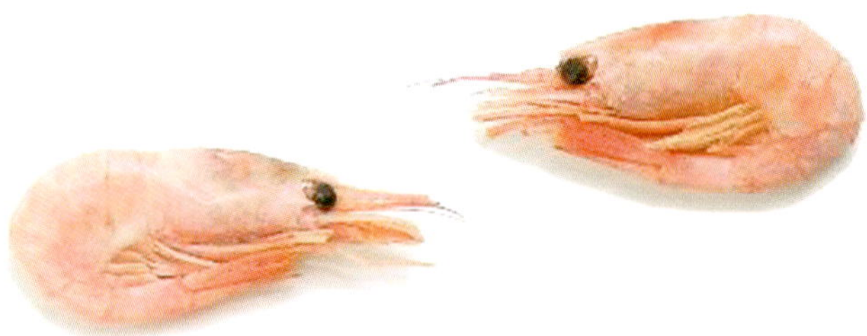

Prawns are an excellent low-calorie choice, and they are a rich source of protein, vitamins and minerals.

Food	Quantity	Glycaemic index	Fat	Protein	Fibre	Calories
Fruit						
Apple	1 medium	L	0	0.5	2	45
Apricot	3	M	0	1.5	2	30
Banana	1 small	M	0.5	1	1	90
Berries, fresh	100 g	L	0	0.5	1	30
Dried fruit	50 g	M	0	0.5	4	80
Grapefruit	half	L	0	0.5	1	30
Melon	slice	M	0	0.5	1	50
Nectarine, peach	1 medium	L	0	0.5	1	35
Orange	1 medium	L	0	1.5	3	50

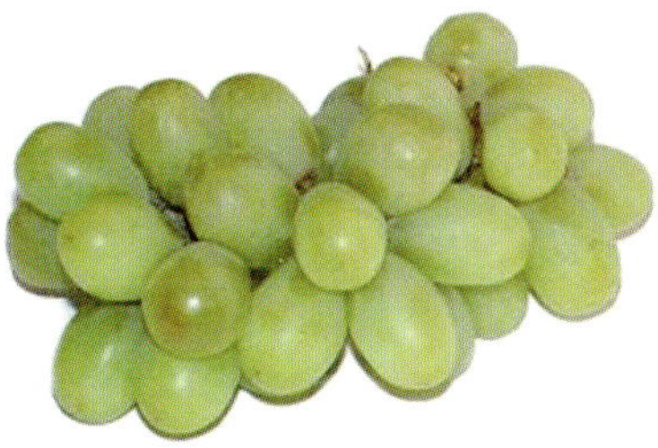

Fruit is easily digested and has many health benefits.

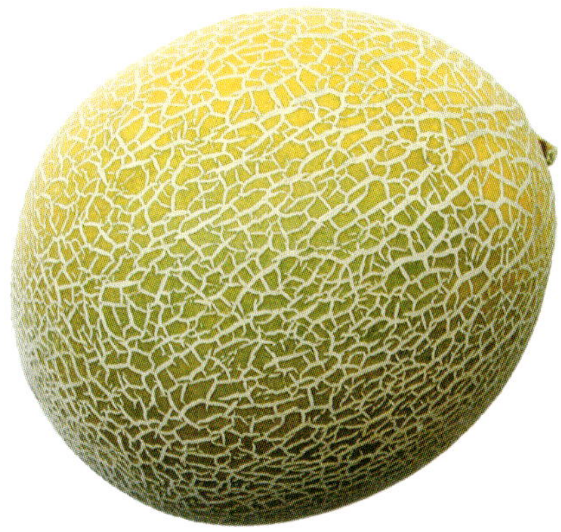

Food	Quantity	Glycaemic index	Fat	Protein	Fibre	Calories
Vegetables						
Aubergine	100 g	L	0	0.5	2	75
Avocado	1/2 medium	L	15	2	3.5	150
Beans	100 g	L	0.5	6	4	100
Beetroot	small	L	0	0.5	0.5	25
Broccoli	100 g	L	0	1.5	2.5	25
Cabbage	50 g	L	0	1	1	7
Carrot	50 g	L	0	0.5	1	12

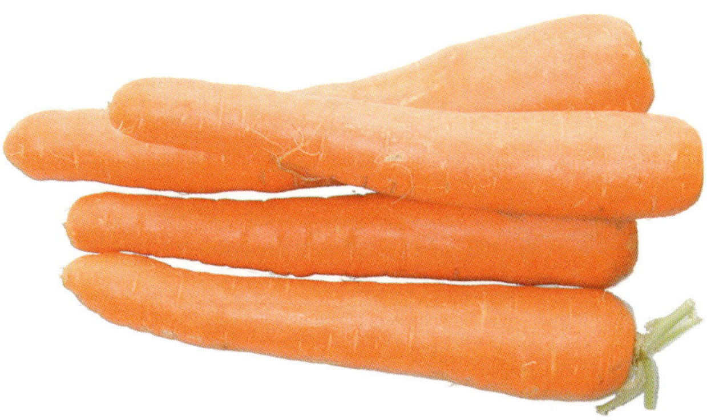

Carrots are high in beta-carotene (providing vitamin A value) and cooking carrots actually enhances the digestibility of the beta-carotene.

Food	Quantity	Glycaemic index	Fat	Protein	Fibre	Calories
Vegetables *(continued)*						
Cauliflower	100 g	L	0	1	1.5	20
Green beans	100 g	L	0	1.5	2.5	20
Onions	medium	L	0	1	1.4	30
Peas	100 g	L	0	3.5	6	60
Peppers	100 g	L	0	1	2.5	30
Potatoes, new	3	M	0	1.5	3	100
Soyabean	100 g	L	7	8	6	120
Spinach	50 g cooked	L	0	1	1	10
Squash, butternut	100 g	M	0	1	1.5	30
Sweetcorn	100 g	M	0.5	2.5	1.5	95
Tofu	100 g	L	4	8	0	70
Tomato	medium	L	0	1	1	15

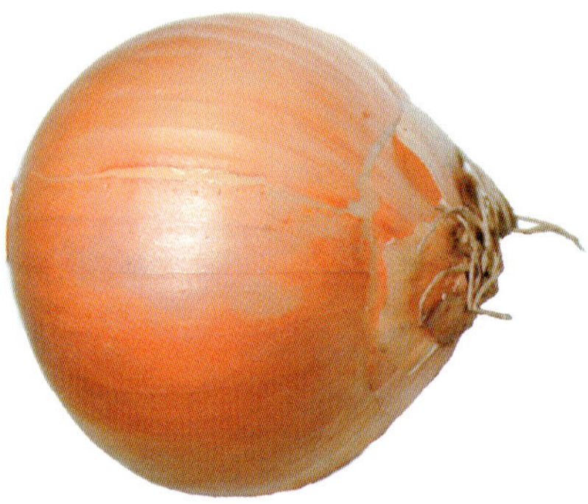

Eating raw onions can help to increase your high-density lipoprotein cholesterol (HDL) levels. This good type of cholesterol can help to keep blood pressure low, so reducing the risk of cardiovascular disease and stroke.

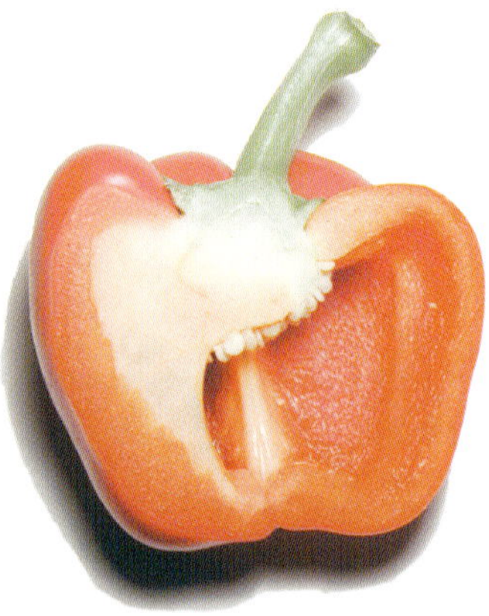

Peppers are low in calories and are especially rich in vitamins A and C. Surprisingly, a pepper contains three to four times more vitamin C than an orange. They do not contain any fat.

Food	Quantity	Glycaemic index	Fat	Protein	Fibre	Calories
Cereal, Nuts, Pulses						
Barley	50 g raw	L	1	2	1	140
Chickpeas	100 g	L	3	5	4	110
Lentils	100 g	L	0.5	8	2	100
Oats	50 g raw	L	1	4	3	140
Pasta, wholegrain	100 g	L	1	5	4	120
Rice, brown, basmati	100 g	M	0	3.5	1	200
Walnuts	2 tbsp	L	8	2	1	80
Wild rice	100 g	M	0	3	1	100

BREAKFASTS

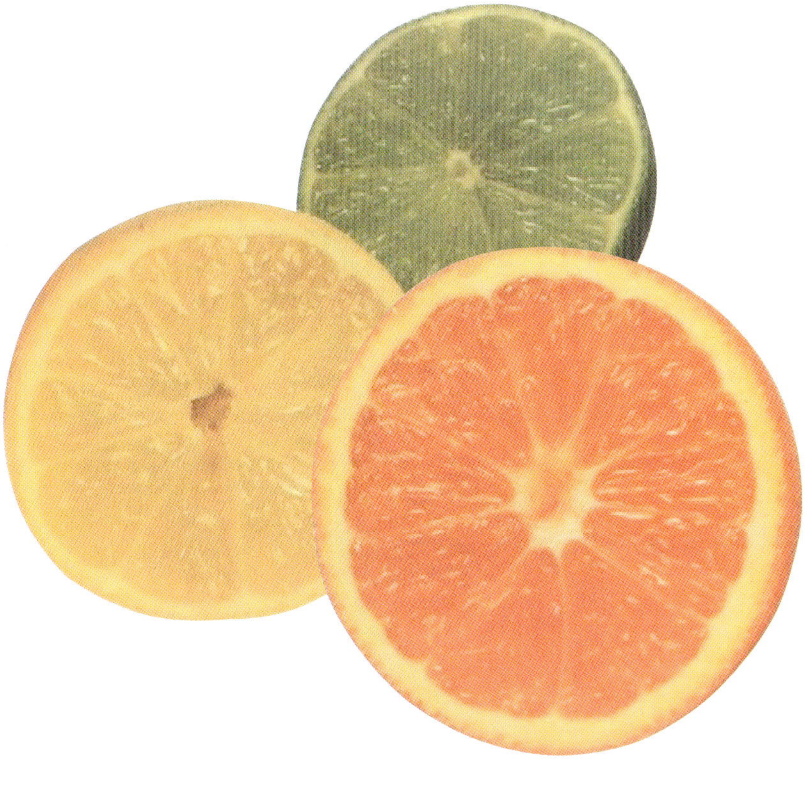

APPLE AND DATE PORRIDGE

SERVES **4**

What better way to start the day than with a healthy, and filling, bowl of porridge. The apple and dates give the porridge an enjoyable sweetness, which can also be achieved with a variety of fruits.

90 g whole rolled porridge oats
15 g bran
450 ml semi-skimmed milk
300 ml water
2 green eating apples, cored and chopped
75 g dried dates, stoned and chopped
2 tbsp dark brown muscovado sugar

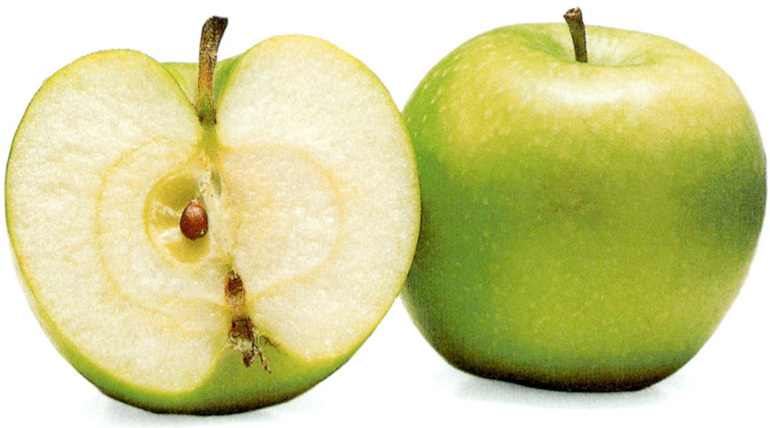

1 Mix the porridge oats, bran, milk and water together in a saucepan.

2 Bring to the boil, stirring occasionally, then simmer for 6 minutes, stirring 3–4 times.

3 Stir in the apple and dates and simmer for a further 3–4 minutes, stirring occasionally.

4 Stir in half the sugar and spoon into 4 individual serving bowls. Sprinkle with the remaining sugar and serve.

NUTRITIONAL VALUES

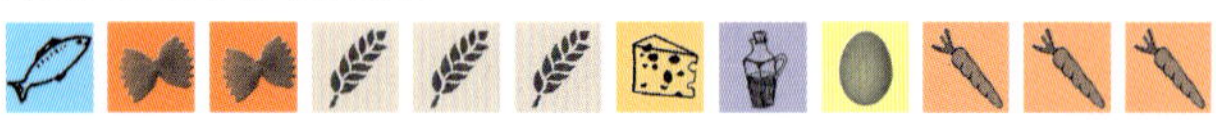

GRAPE AND ORANGE GRANOLA

SERVES **4**

This breakfast gives you a healthy start to the day, and has a great variety of texture and flavour.

2 tbsp light olive oil
2 tbsp malt extract
2 tbsp clear honey
75 g rolled oats
50 g jumbo oats
25 g barley flakes
25 g desiccated coconut
15 g sesame seeds
25 g sunflower seeds
25 g mixed nuts, chopped
$^1/_2$ tsp ground mixed spice
$^1/_2$ tsp ground cinnamon

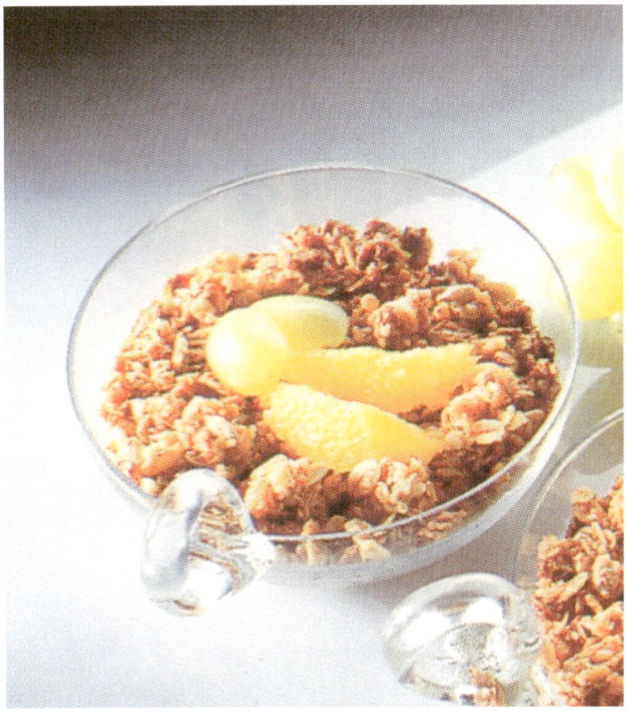

TO SERVE

150 g green seedless grapes, halved
2 oranges, segmented
skimmed milk or low-fat natural yoghurt

1. Mix the oil, malt and honey together in a saucepan and heat gently until runny.
2. Stir the oats, barley flakes, coconut, sesame and sunflower seeds, nuts and spices into the honey mix.
3. Spread evenly over a large baking tray or roasting pan and bake in a preheated oven at 190°C/gas mark 5 for 20–25 minutes, until golden and crisp. Stir 3–4 times to avoid over-browning on the top surface.
4. Leave to cool, then store in an airtight container until required.
5. To serve, place in individual bowls and arrange the grapes and orange segments on top. Serve with skimmed milk or natural low fat yoghurt as required.

NUTRITIONAL VALUES

BREAKFAST SALAD

SERVES **4–6**

In Israel, breakfast is salad. Most meals in Israel include salad: crisp, crunchy and juicy with a wide variety of ingredients, which always include green, yellow and red peppers, and hot peppers, too, if you wish.

1 cucumber, unpeeled and diced
1 each: green, red, yellow or orange pepper, diced
6 ripe tomatoes, diced
2 tbsp each: fresh chopped parsley, coriander, dill (optional) and mint (optional)
3 cloves garlic, chopped
3 spring onions, sliced thin
salt substitute (see page 18)
½ to 1 hot chilli, chopped (optional)
3–4 tbsp extra virgin olive oil
juice of 1–1½ lemons

1 Combine all the ingredients and chill until ready to serve.

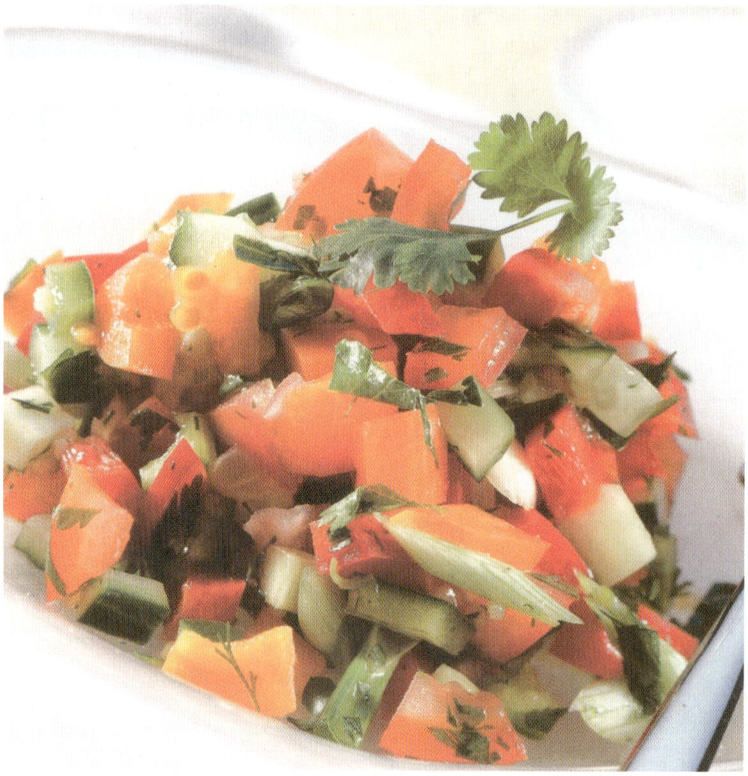

NUTRITIONAL VALUES

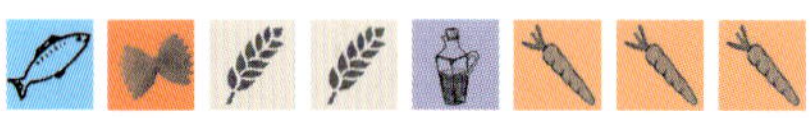

APRICOT YOGHURT CRUNCH

SERVES **4**

A variation on a Scottish dish, the crunchy porridge oats, spicy yoghurt, and lightly poached fruit make an attractive morning dish.

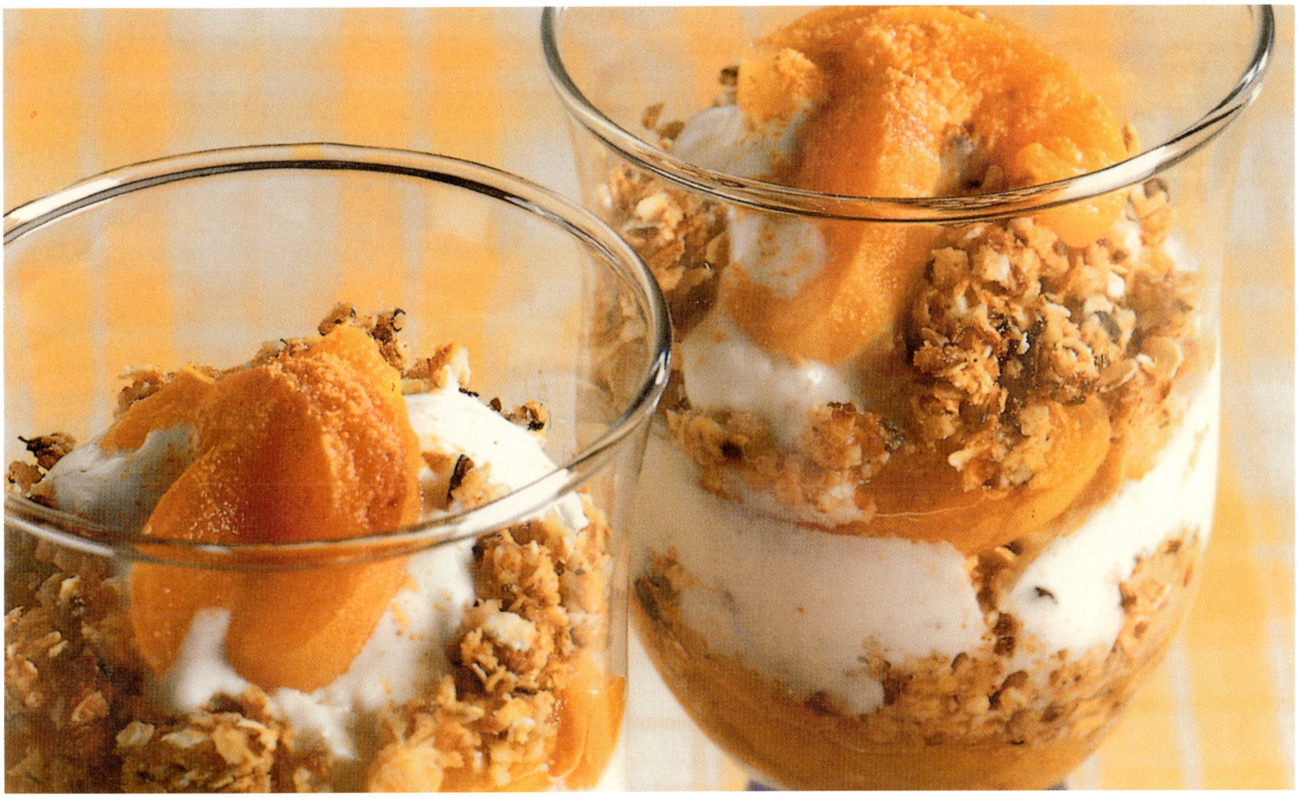

275 g apricots, pitted
3 tbsp honey
50 g porridge oats, toasted
$^{1}/_{2}$–1 tsp ground ginger
275 g low-fat natural yoghurt

1 Place the apricots in a pan with 150 ml water and 1 tablespoon of the honey. Cook for 5 minutes until softened and drain.

2 Mix the oats and remaining honey in a bowl. Stir the ginger into the yoghurt.

3 Alternately layer the fruit, yoghurt, and oat mixtures into serving glasses. Chill and serve.

NUTRITIONAL VALUES

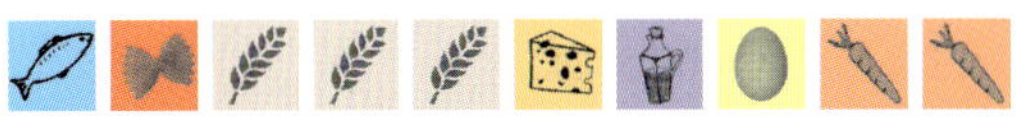

RAISIN BRAN CRUNCH

SERVES **4**

It's important to have a good meal for breakfast, and this is bound to keep you going through to lunchtime.

175 g raisins

450 g bran

170 g oatmeal

12 tbsp sesame seeds (preferably unroasted)

10 tbsp sunflower seeds (unroasted)

250 g less 2 tbsp unsweetened orange juice

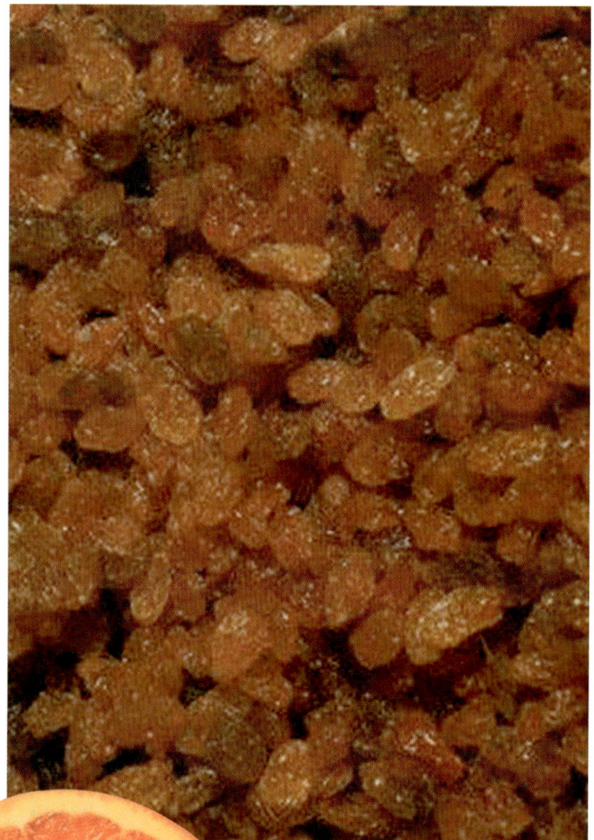

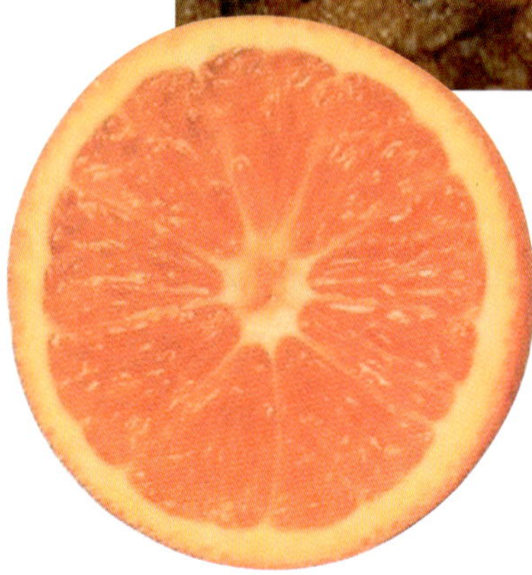

1 Mix the raisins, bran, oatmeal and both types of seeds in a large bowl, then stir in the orange juice.

2 Preheat the oven to 160°C/gas mark 3.

3 Lightly grease a large roasting pan. Stir the mixture thoroughly, then turn it into the pan – do not press it down. Bake for about 2 hours, turning and stirring occasionally, until well browned, crisp and dry.

4 Allow to cool in the pan, then break the mixture up into small lumps and store them in an airtight container.

5 Serve with milk.

NUTRITIONAL VALUES

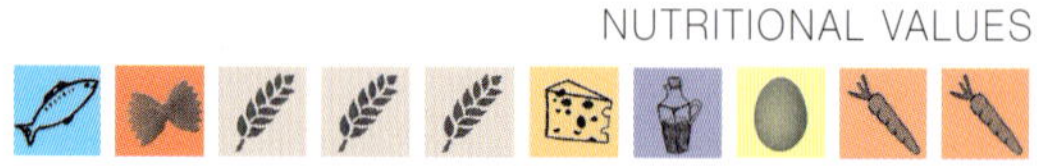

LIGHT MEALS

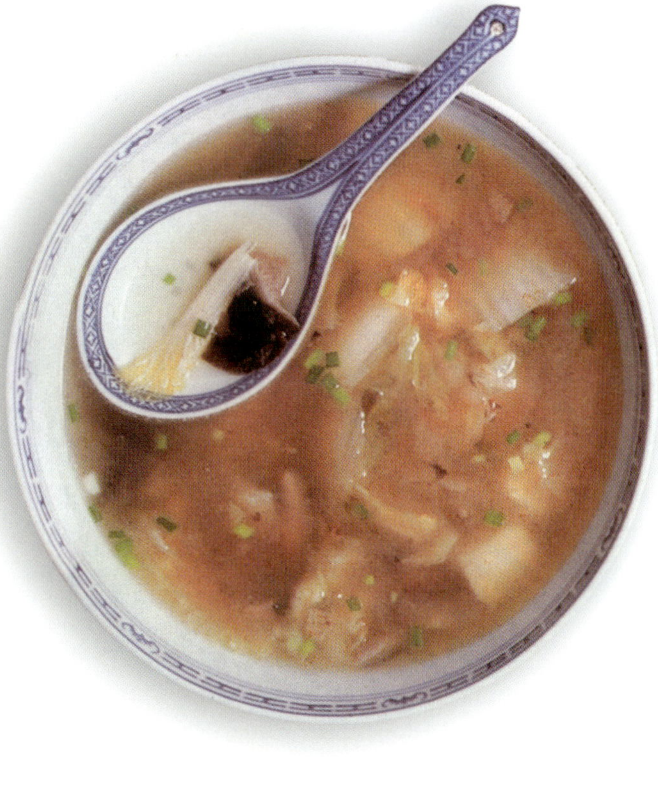

CHESTNUT, DATE AND APPLE SALAD

SERVES **6**

This meal contains a great variety of fruits and vegetables that keeps you going through the day.

450 g chestnuts, shelled and peeled
750 ml chicken stock
1 bay leaf
225 g pitted dates, halved
1 large red-skinned apple
1 large green-skinned apple
1 medium-size carrot, thinly sliced
3 shallots, sliced diagonally
1 garlic clove, minced
2 tbsp fresh lemon juice
$1\frac{1}{2}$ tsp curry powder
freshly ground black pepper to taste
6 tbsp olive oil

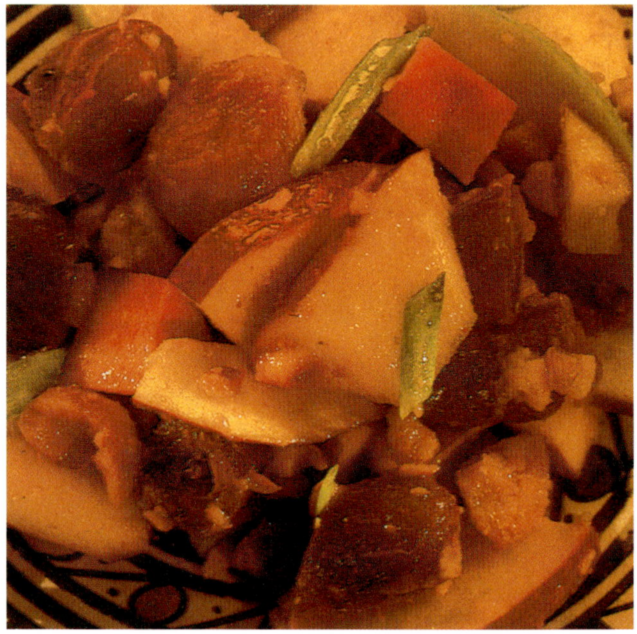

1 Place the chestnuts in a small saucepan with the stock and bay leaf. Bring to a simmer, cover, and continue to simmer for 30–40 minutes or until the chestnuts are tender. Keep the heat low so the chestnuts don't fall apart. Allow them to cool in the cooking liquid. (Cooling can be hastened by setting the pan in a sink filled with 2.5–5 cm of cold water.)

2 Drain the chestnuts and remove the bay leaf.

3 In a salad or mixing bowl, combine the chestnuts and dates. Without peeling, quarter, core and slice the apples and add them to the bowl along with the carrot and shallots.

4 In a small bowl, whisk together the garlic, lemon juice, curry powder and pepper. Whisk in the olive oil and toss with the salad ingredients. Serve at once.

NUTRITIONAL VALUES

ONION, ORANGE AND TOMATO SALAD

SERVES **4**

A great salad to serve with fish dishes. The vinaigrette recipe given here is the perfect complement to this dish.

- 2 handfuls rocket
- 2 handfuls watercress
- 2 heads Belgian chicory, trimmed and finely sliced
- 1 orange, peeled and divided into segments
- 4 ripe tomatoes, cut into wedges
- 6 spring onions, trimmed and finely chopped
- freshly ground black pepper

VINAIGRETTE

- 4 tbsp olive oil
- 1 tbsp white wine vinegar
- 1 tbsp Dijon mustard
- freshly ground black pepper, and lemon juice to taste

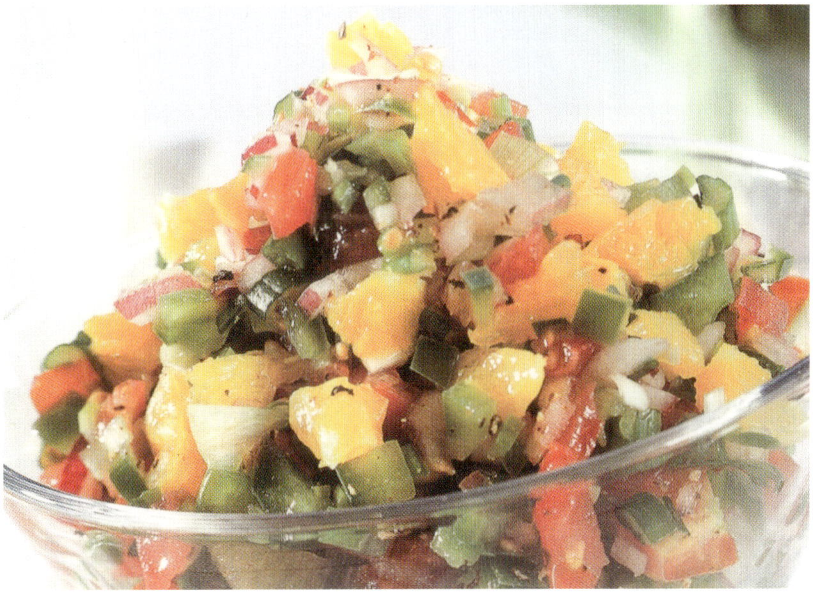

1 Arrange the rocket, watercress and Belgian chicory in a large bowl. Cut the orange segments in half, remove any seeds, then toss them in with the tomatoes and spring onions. Season lightly.

2 Whisk all the vinaigrette ingredients together until thoroughly blended. Spoon over the salad, mix, and serve.

NUTRITIONAL VALUES

CABBAGE WITH PEAS

SERVES **4**

This meal can be served on its own, or as a side dish as an accompaniment to lean meat.

- 3 tbsp olive oil
- 2 bay leaves
- 3/4 tsp whole cumin seeds
- 700 g cabbage, finely shredded
- 1 tsp ground turmeric
- 1/2 tsp chilli powder
- 1 1/2 tsp ground cumin
- 1 tsp ground coriander
- 2 tomatoes, chopped
- 100 g peas

NUTRITIONAL VALUES

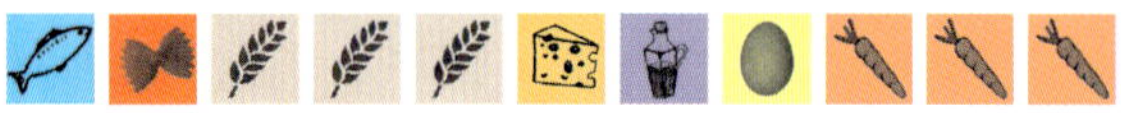

1 Heat the oil in a karai over medium–high heat and add the bay leaves and the cumin seeds. Let them sizzle for a few seconds.

2 Add the cabbage and stir for 2–3 minutes.

3 Add the turmeric, chilli, cumin, coriander and tomatoes, and mix with the cabbage.

4 Lower the heat, cover and cook for 15 minutes. Add the peas and cover again. Continue to cook for a further 15 minutes, stirring occasionally.

5 Remove the cover, turn heat up to medium–high and, stirring continuously, cook until it is dry.

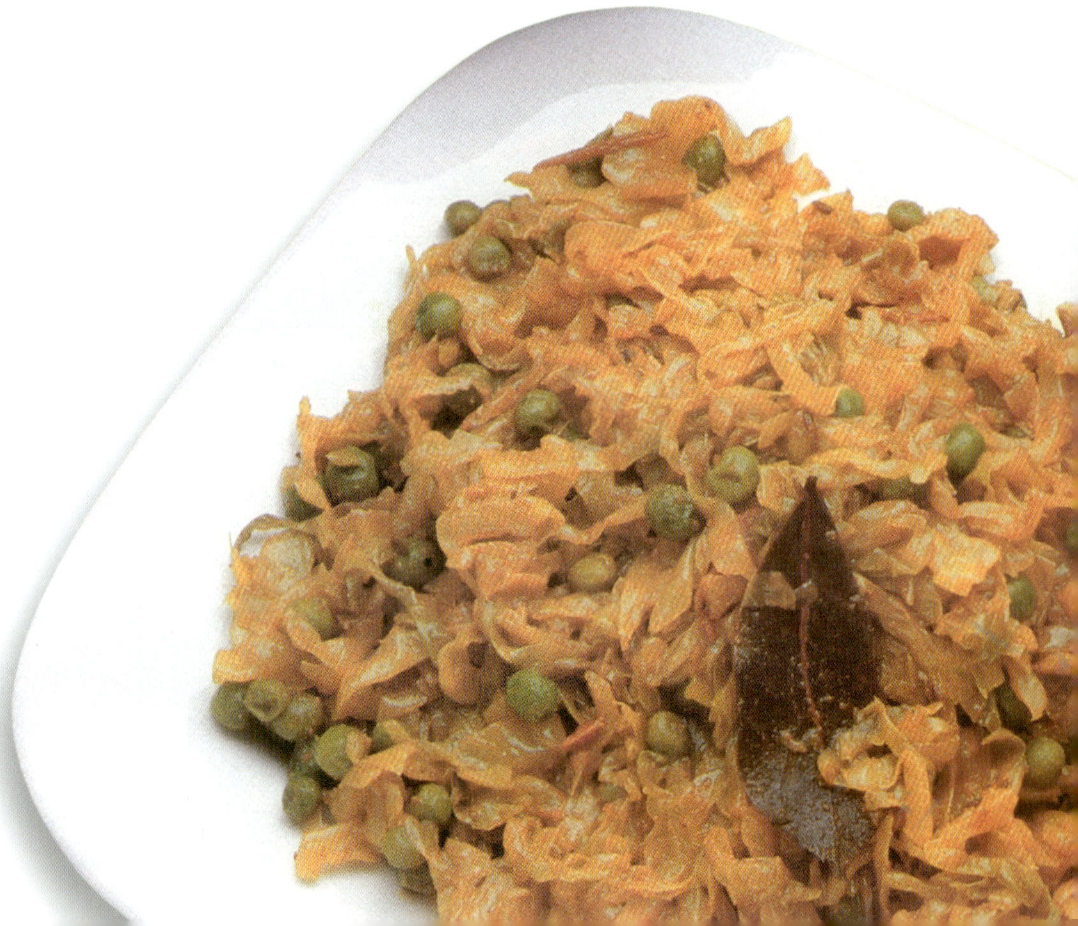

SALAD OF BEETROOT, LAMB'S LETTUCE AND CLEMENTINES

SERVES **4**

A fantastic dish that has heaps of colour, which will impress all your dinner guests.

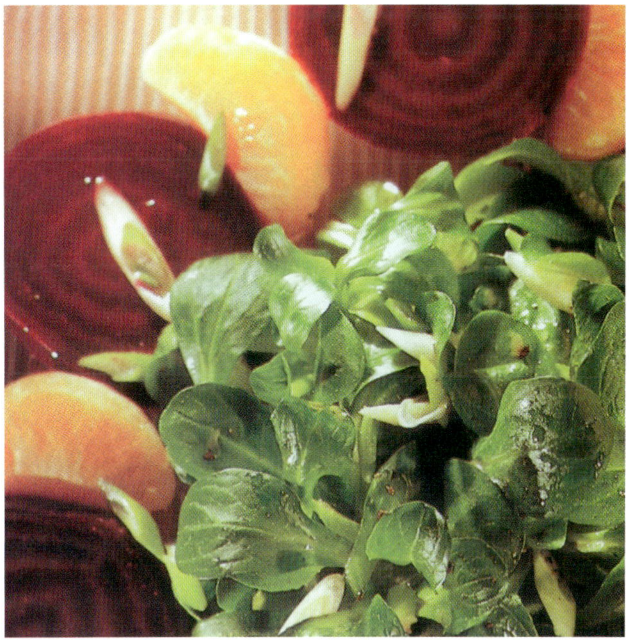

SALAD

4 beetroots, each 5 cm in diameter

4 handfuls lamb's lettuce, washed and roots trimmed

4 clementines, peeled, segmented and pith removed

2 spring onions thinly sliced

VINAIGRETTE

1 tbsp balsamic vinegar

1 tbsp lemon juice

1 tsp Dijon mustard

freshly ground black pepper

4 tbsp good quality virgin olive oil

1 Top and tail the beetroots, leaving 5 cm of stalk and root attached. Drop them into boiling water and boil for 25–30 minutes, or until just tender. Then plunge them into a basin of cold water until cool. Cut off the ends and slice crossways into 3 mm thick slices.

2 Arrange the beetroot slices and clementine segments around 4 serving plates. Pile the lamb's lettuce in the centre of each plate. Scatter the spring onions over each salad.

3 In a small bowl, combine the vinegar, lemon juice, mustard and pepper to taste. Whisk, adding the oil in a stream. When all the oil has been incorporated, drizzle the vinaigrette over the salads and serve.

NUTRITIONAL VALUES

STAR FRUIT AND ROCKET SALAD WITH RASPBERRY VINEGAR DRESSING

SERVES **4**

Rocket has a strong, very distinctive flavour which is excellent when balanced with sweet salad greens such as iceberg or Romaine lettuce, but do not be tempted to add too much rocket or cut it too coarsely as it will overpower the other delicate ingredients, especially the star fruit.

½ iceberg lettuce, shredded
12 medium rocket leaves, finely shredded
3 spring onions or green onions, chopped
2 star fruit, sliced and quartered

FOR THE DRESSING

3 tbsp raspberry vinegar
1 tsp caster sugar
freshly ground black pepper
8 tbsp olive oil

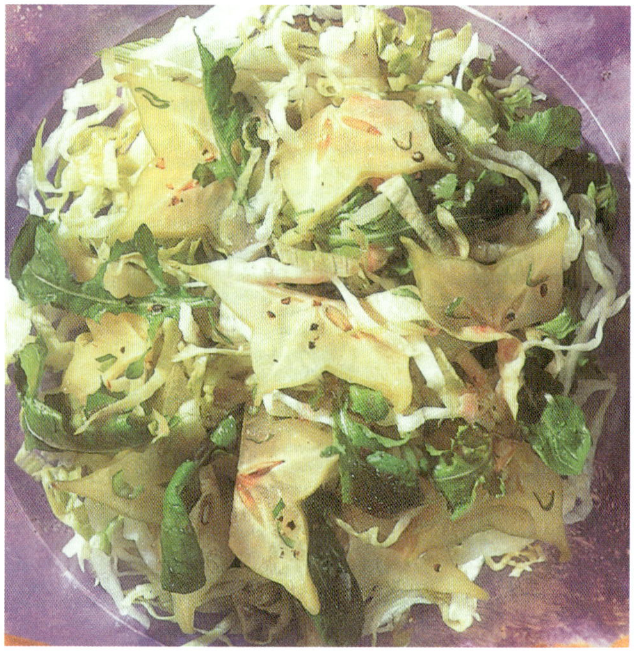

NUTRITIONAL VALUES

1 Toss the lettuce, rocket and spring onions together in a salad bowl. Next make the dressing: place the vinegar in a basin and whisk in the caster sugar with plenty of seasoning. Continue whisking until the sugar has dissolved. Slowly add the olive oil, whisking all the time to combine the ingredients well.

2 Add the star fruit to the salad. Pour the dressing over the mix lightly. Serve at once. Do not leave the star fruit to stand for any length of time once it is cut as it dries on the surface and tends to discolour slightly around the edges.

FLAGEOLET BEANS WITH SPINACH

SERVES **4**

This no-fuss, no-meat, light meal is ideal for summer days when spare time is best spent outdoors rather than slaving for hours in a hot kitchen.

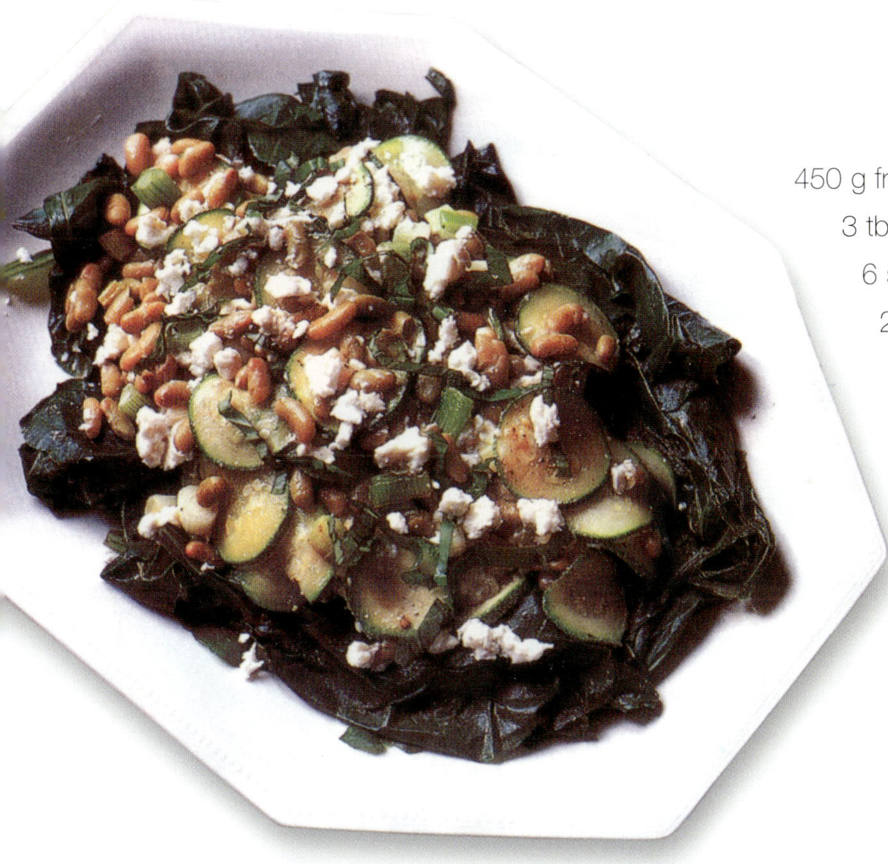

- 450 g fresh spinach, trimmed and washed
- 3 tbsp olive oil
- 6 spring onions, chopped
- 2 x 425 g cans flageolet beans, drained
- 2 small courgettes, trimmed and thinly sliced
- 2 tbsp chopped fresh mint
- several large basil sprigs, leaves shredded
- 225 g feta cheese, crumbled
- salt substitute (see page 18) and freshly ground black pepper

1 Press all the spinach leaves into a large saucepan while still dripping wet. Put a lid on the pan and place it over high heat. Cook, shaking the pan often, for about 5 minutes, or until the spinach has wilted and shrunk.

2 Stir the leaves, cover and cook for a further 2 minutes or so, until tender. Drain well, then replace the spinach in the pan and add 1 tablespoon of the oil. Cover and leave over low heat to keep hot.

3 Heat the remaining oil, then stir-fry the scallions, flageolet beans, and courgettes for 5 minutes, until the courgettes are just cooked. Spoon the spinach on to 1 large or 4 individual serving plates. Toss the mint, basil and feta into the vegetables, and add seasoning to taste.

4 Spoon the vegetables over the spinach and then serve the dish at once.

NUTRITIONAL VALUES

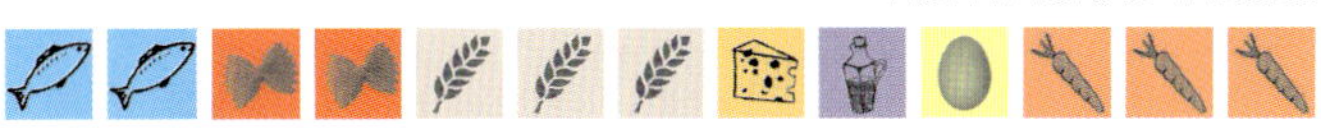

SPINACH WITH COTTAGE CHEESE

SERVES **4**

A quick and easy meal to cook, that produces a dish full of flavour.

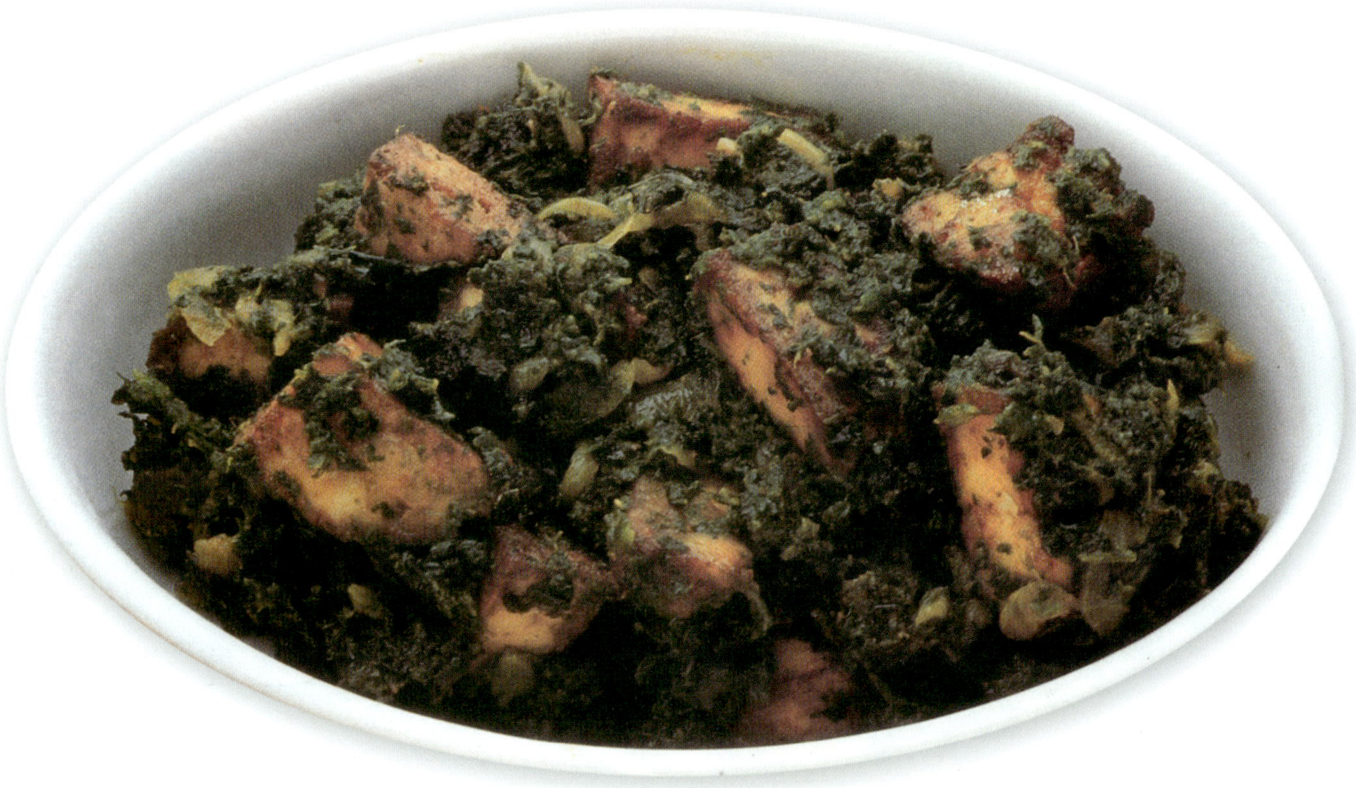

4 tbsp olive oil

75 g panir, drained and cut into 1 cm cubes

1 large onion, finely sliced

4 cloves garlic, crushed

1 cm root ginger, grated

350 g frozen spinach, chopped

$^1/_2$ tsp ground turmeric

$^1/_3$ tsp chilli powder

1 tsp ground coriander

1. Heat oil in a karai over medium–high heat and fry the panir until brown. Set aside.
2. Add the onion, garlic and ginger in the remaining oil and fry until golden.
3. Add the spinach, turmeric, chilli coriander and fry for 2–3 minutes.
4. Lower the heat to medium, cover and cook for a further 10 minutes.
5. Add the fried panir and, stirring constantly, cook until dry.

NUTRITIONAL VALUES

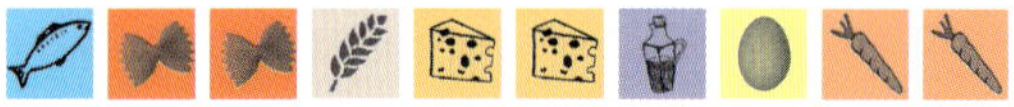

DOLCELATTE AND SPINACH FILO TART

SERVES **4**

This is a delicious tart, suitable for eating hot, warm or cold. Serve it as a light starter or add a green salad or vegetables and serve it as a more substantial meal.

1 tbsp olive oil
4 shallots, finely chopped
4 garlic cloves, crushed
200 g fresh spinach, washed and stems removed
180 g Dolcelatte cheese, crumbled
2 eggs, lightly beaten
5 tbsp low-fat crème fraîche
freshly ground black pepper
20 g butter, melted
about 60 g filo pastry sheets

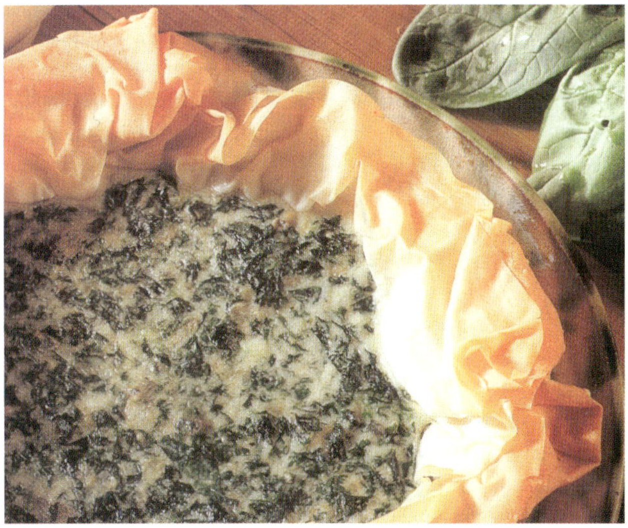

1 Preheat the oven to 190°C/gas mark 5. Heat the oil in a large saucepan and sauté the shallots and garlic very gently until soft.

2 Meanwhile, place the spinach in a large pan (with no water), cover and cook for a few minutes until it has wilted. Once cooked, drain the spinach in a sieve, squeeze out as much of the liquid as possible, and roughly chop it.

3 Stir the cheese into the shallots and cook for a further minute until the cheese has melted slightly. Remove from the heat and stir in the spinach. Beat together the eggs and crème fraîche, season with pepper and add to the spinach mixture, mixing well.

4 Lightly grease an 18 cm diameter, $2^{1}/_{2}$ cm deep, loose-bottomed tart tin with some of the melted butter. Cut the pastry into 8 pieces, approximately 20 x 28 cm. (If the pastry you are using does not match these dimensions, simply cut it as neatly as possible and continue as described, using a few extra sheets if necessary.)

5 Take one sheet of pastry and brush it with melted butter. Lay it across half the tin, leaving the edges hanging over the sides of the dish. Brush a second piece of pastry with butter and use it to cover the other half of the tin. Rotate the tin through 90° and repeat with 2 more pieces of pastry, brushing each one with butter. Turn the tin twice more, 90° each time, and repeat with the final 4 pieces of pastry.

6 Place the tart on a baking sheet. Spoon the spinach mixture into the tin and scrunch the edges of the pastry together. Bake in the oven for 20 minutes, until the pastry is golden and the filling is set.

7 To serve, carefully remove the tart from the tin and serve accompanied by a green salad or vegetables.

NUTRITIONAL VALUES

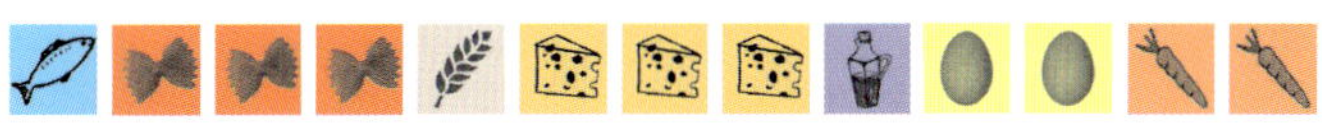

CHINESE CABBAGE SOUP

SERVES **4**

Most Chinese dishes are quick and easy to make and have great combinations of flavours, and this soup is no exception.

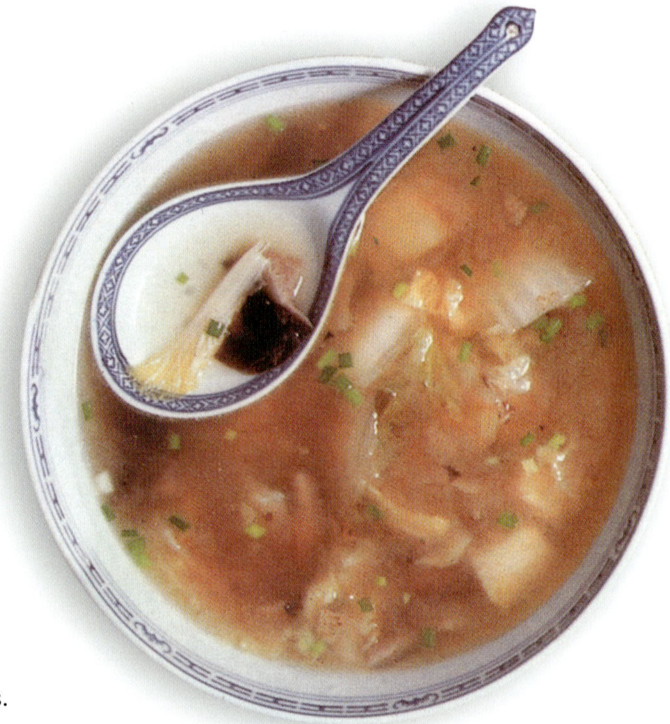

250 g Chinese cabbage

3–4 dried Chinese mushrooms, soaked in warm water for 30 minutes

2 tbsp olive oil

2 tsp salt substitute (see page 18)

1 tbsp rice wine or dry sherry

900 g water

1 tsp sesame seed oil

1 Wash the cabbage and cut it into thin slices. Squeeze dry the soaked mushrooms. Discard the hard stalks and cut the mushrooms into small pieces. Reserve the water in which the mushrooms have been soaked for use later.

2 Heat a wok or large pan until hot, add the olive oil and wait for it to smoke. Add the cabbage and mushrooms. Stir a few times and then add the salt substitute, wine, water and the water in which the mushrooms have been soaked. Bring to the boil, add the sesame seed oil and serve.

NUTRITIONAL VALUES

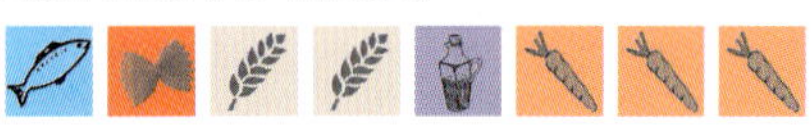

FATTOUSH

SERVES **4**

This salad of stale bread and salad vegetables from Lebanon, characteristically dressed with lots of olive oil and lemon, is very refreshing.

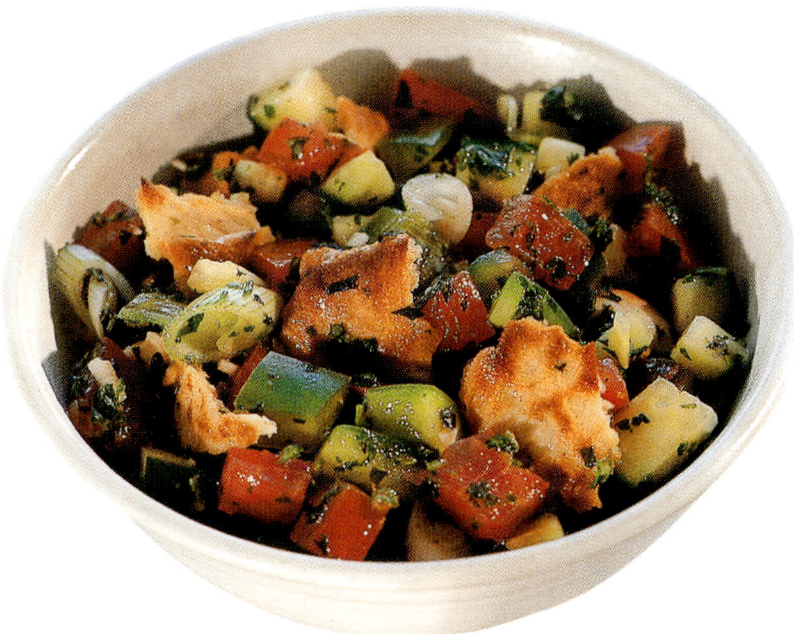

1 large or 2 small cucumbers, diced
3 ripe tomatoes, diced
1 green pepper, diced
25 g (about 8 tbsp) each: fresh mint, fresh chopped coriander, fresh chopped parsley
3 spring onions, thinly sliced
3 garlic cloves
75 ml extra virgin olive oil
juice of 3 lemons
1 tsp sumac
3–4 pitta breads, stale and lightly toasted, then broken into pieces

1 Combine the cucumbers, tomatoes, pepper, mint, coriander, parsley, spring onions, garlic, olive oil, lemon juice and sumac. Chill for at least 1 hour. Just before serving, toss with the broken pitta breads.

NUTRITIONAL VALUES

CHILLI-SPICED BROCCOLI

SERVES **4**

This dish is from southern Italy. Use a chilli that is not too hot, with just enough bite to make it 'all' arrabbiata' *(angry), the term given in Italy to chilli-spiced dishes. The spicy broccoli can be mixed into spaghetti.*

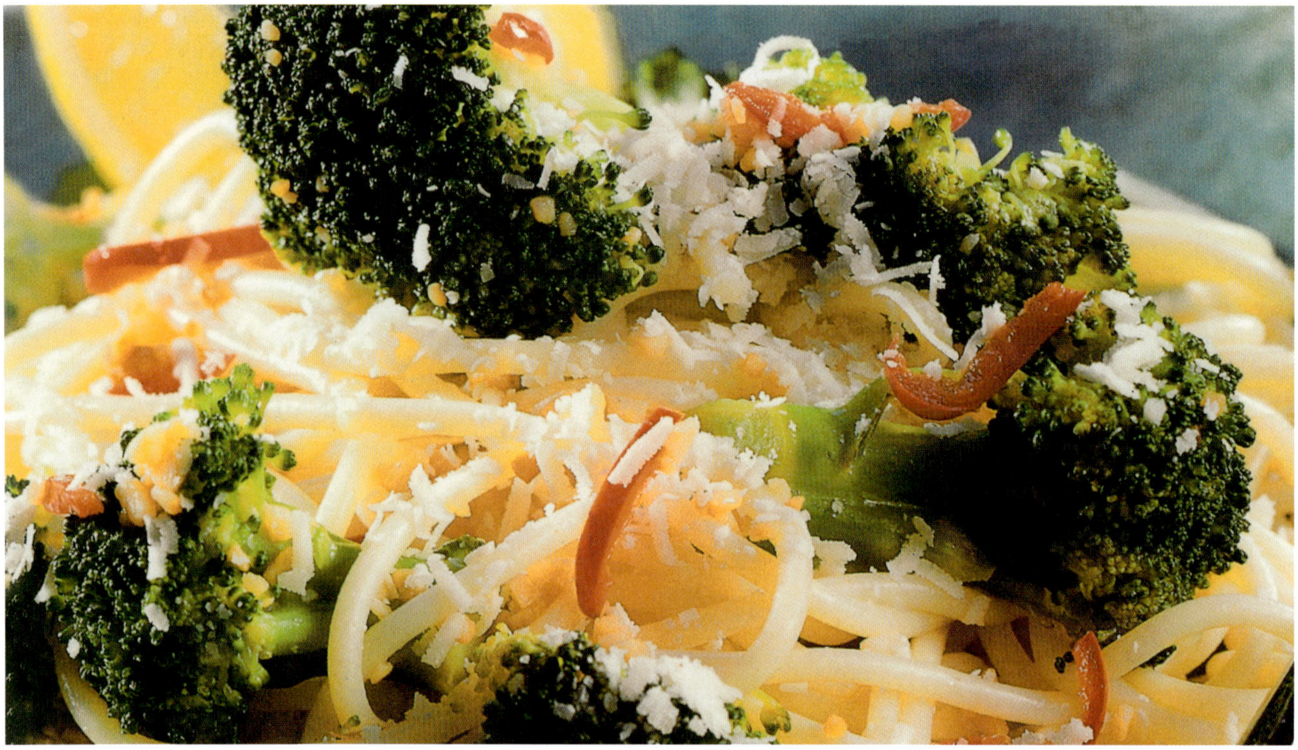

1 large or 2 medium-sized bunches broccoli, broken into florets, the stems peeled and cut into bite-sized pieces
2 tbsp extra virgin olive oil
3–5 cloves garlic, sliced thin
1 medium-hot or mild fresh red chilli, or more as desired, thinly sliced, or chopped
juice of $^1/_4$–$^1/_2$ lemon or to taste
grated Parmesan cheese (optional)

NUTRITIONAL VALUES

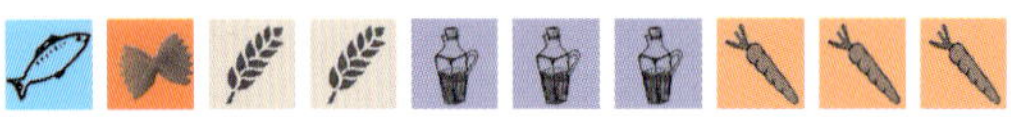

1 Blanch the broccoli in boiling water. Cook for only a minute or two, or until the broccoli is crisp-tender and bright green. Remove from the heat, rinse well in cold water, and dry.

2 In a wok or large frying pan heat the olive oil, garlic, and chilli, and warm through, then add the broccoli and cook together for a few minutes to mix the flavours. Squeeze the lemon juice over the vegetables and remove from the heat.

3 Serve the broccoli and red chillies hot, with a grating of Parmesan cheese, if wished, or at room temperature, with a little more lemon juice drizzled over the top.

MINTED PEPPER SALAD

SERVES **4**

Make this cool, light and colourful salad for a summer lunch or picnic, but do not drizzle over the olive oil until ready to serve.

350 g dried macaroni

dash of olive oil, plus extra for drizzling

1 yellow pepper, cored, deseeded and cut into diamonds

1 green pepper cored, deseeded and cut into diamonds

350 g can artichoke hearts, drained and quartered

15 cm piece of cucumber, sliced

handful of mint leaves

freshly ground black pepper

100 g freshly grated Parmesan cheese

1. Bring a saucepan of water to the boil, and add the macaroni with a dash of olive oil.
2. Cook for 10 minutes, until tender. Drain, rinse, then place in a mixing bowl.
3. Mix the remaining ingredients into the pasta. Drizzle some olive oil over the salad, then serve.

NUTRITIONAL VALUES

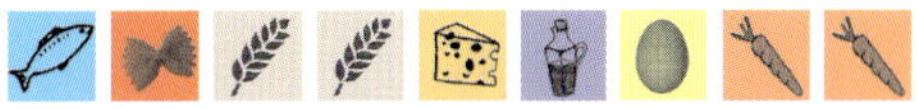

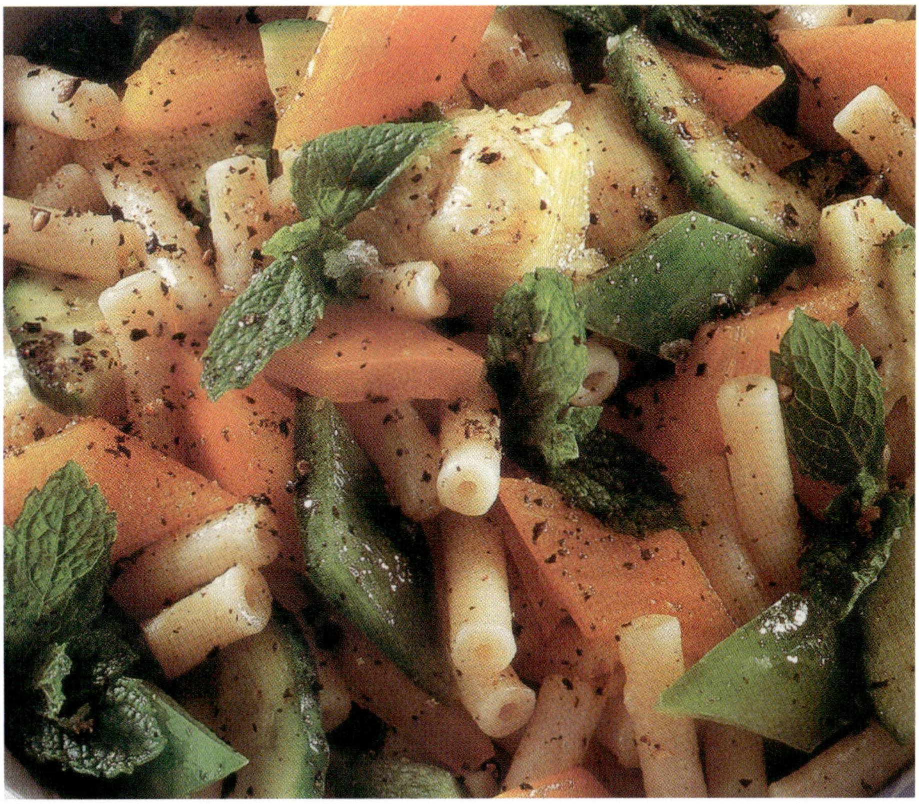

WARM PASTA SALAD

SERVES **4**

This salad combines the saltiness of green olives, the crunch of walnuts and the goodness of fresh vegetables. The flavours are enhanced when it is served warm, but if you have cold leftovers, add a splash of vinaigrette for flavour.

225 g pasta shapes
100 g asparagus
4 tbsp extra virgin olive oil
4 tbsp freshly grated Parmesan cheese plus extra for sprinkling
1 courgette, finely shredded
4 spring onions, sliced
25 g walnuts, chopped
8 green olives, stoned
freshly ground black pepper

NUTRITIONAL VALUES

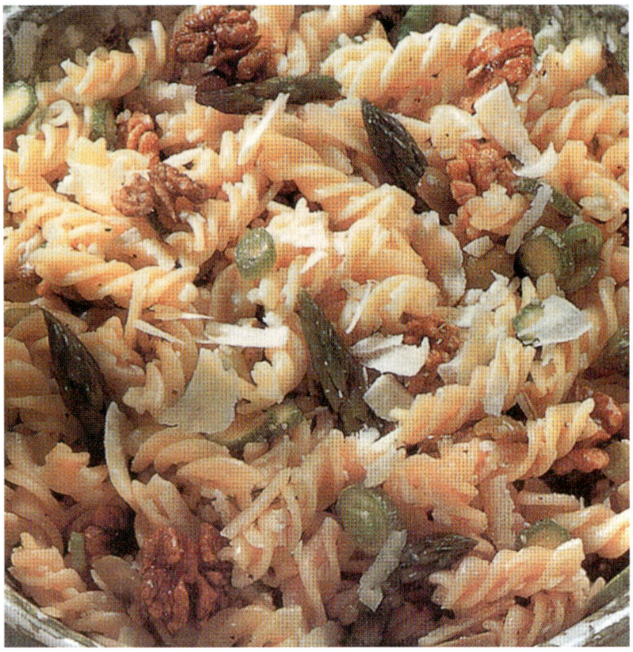

1 Cook the pasta according to directions on the packet. While the pasta is cooking, blanch the asparagus for 2–3 minutes in boiling water. Drain the asparagus, and cut into 2.5 cm pieces.

2 When the pasta is cooked, drain but do not rinse, then put it in a large mixing bowl. Pour olive oil over the pasta, and toss with two forks. Add the Parmesan, and toss again. Stir in the asparagus, courgette, spring onions, walnuts, and green olives. Add pepper to taste. Serve with a sprinkling of Parmesan over the top.

MIXED CABBAGE COLESLAW

SERVES **4–8**

Coleslaw can be a fattening dish, but as long as you use a low-fat yoghurt dressing, this can be a healthy and delicious source of fruits and vegetables.

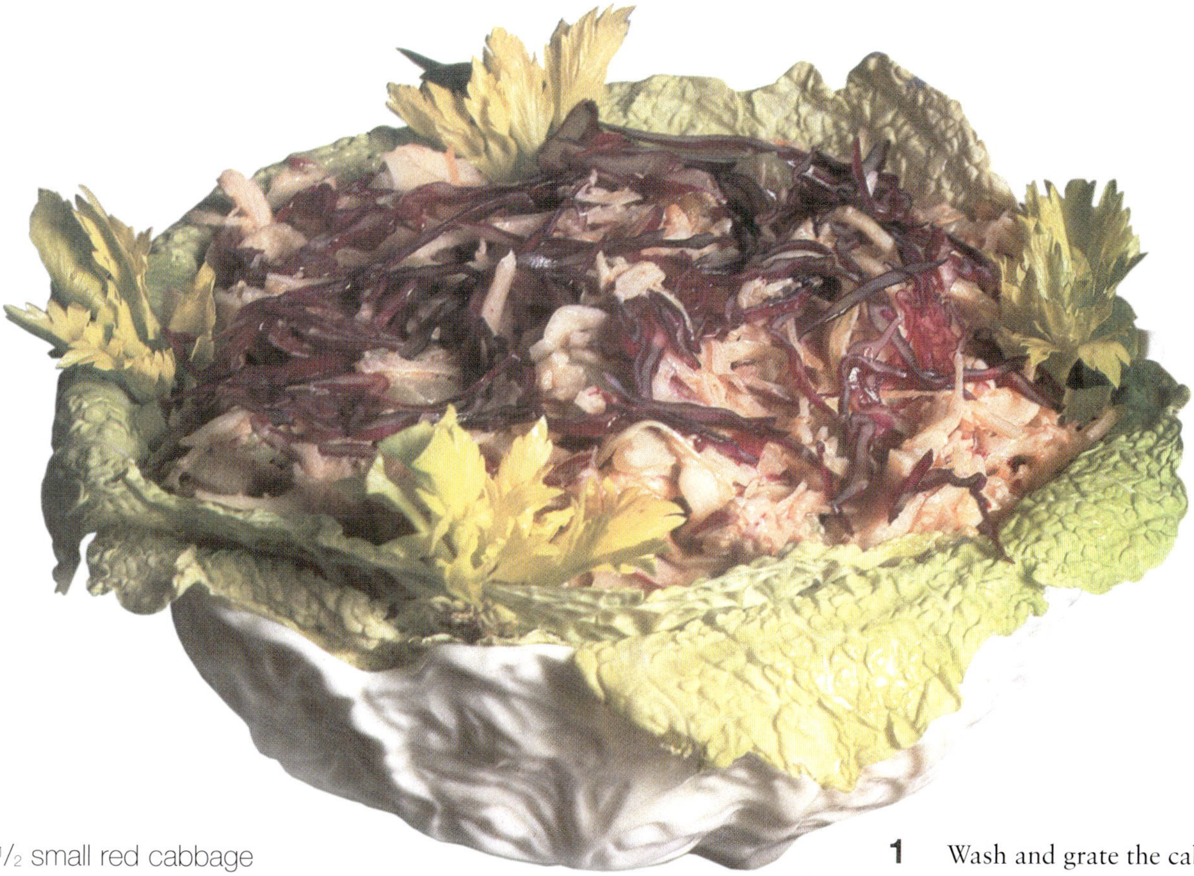

- 1/2 small red cabbage
- 1/2 small white cabbage
- 6 sticks celery, washed
- 2 carrots, grated
- 2 green apples
- 2 tbsp lemon juice
- 1 small onion, peeled
- 50 g chopped walnuts
- 300 ml low-fat yoghurt dressing

NUTRITIONAL VALUES

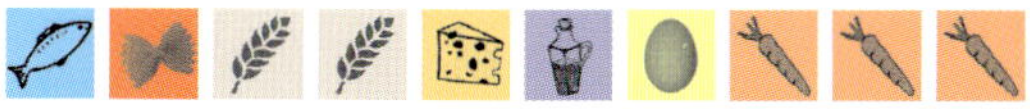

1. Wash and grate the cabbage finely into a bowl.
2. Wash the celery and reserve some leaves for decoration. Remove the strings with a potato peeler and chop finely. Add to the cabbage with the grated carrot and mix well.
3. Wash and dice the apples, sprinkle with lemon juice and add to the cabbage.
4. Slice the onion finely and add to the cabbage mixture with the walnuts. Mix well with the chosen dressing and arrange in a bowl lined with cabbage leaves. Decorate with celery leaves and serve as part of a salad dish or with wholemeal rolls as a snack meal.

FETTUCCINE WITH GARLICKY CREAMED SPINACH

SERVES **4–6**

This tasty recipe is quick and easy to prepare. Serve immediately with plenty of freshly grated Parmesan cheese.

450 g dried fettuccine
dash of olive oil
2 tbsp olive oil
3 cloves garlic, crushed
450 g frozen chopped spinach, thawed and well drained
275 g low-fat crème fraîche
pinch of freshly grated nutmeg
freshly ground black pepper
50 g freshly shredded Parmesan cheese, plus extra to serve

NUTRITIONAL VALUES

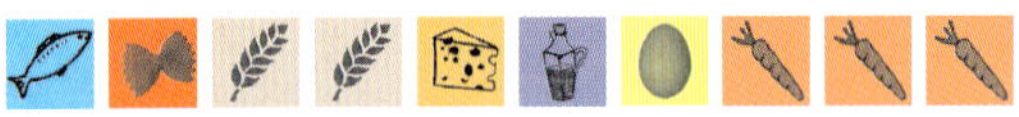

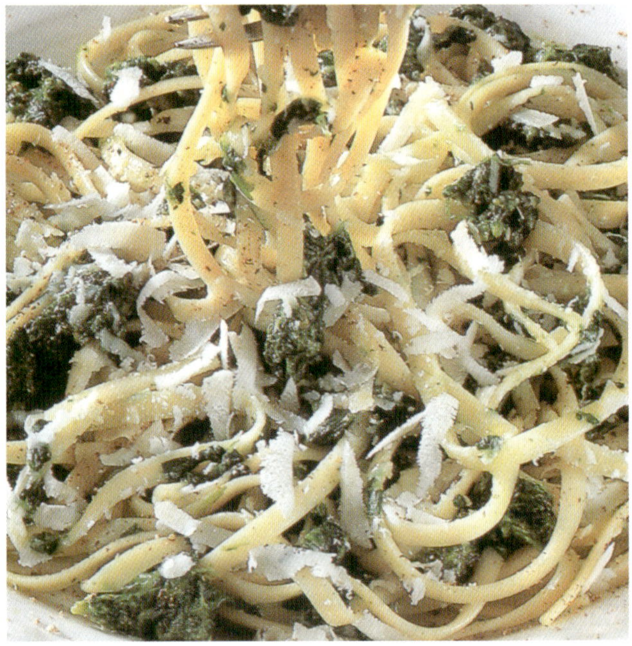

1 Bring a large saucepan of water to the boil and add the fettuccine with a dash of olive oil. Cook for about 8 minutes, stirring occasionally, until tender. Drain and set aside, covered, to keep warm.

2 Sauté the garlic in the olive oil for 1–2 minutes, then add the spinach. Cook over medium heat for about 5 minutes, stirring frequently, until the moisture has evaporated.

3 Add the crème fraîche and nutmeg and season with freshly ground black pepper. Toss in the fettuccine and Parmesan cheese, stir and cook for a final minute. Serve with extra freshly grated Parmesan cheese.

WILTED GREENS WITH FUSILLI

SERVES **4–6**

This quick-to-prepare, nutritious dish is perfect for a light lunch when entertaining friends.

450 g dried fusilli (small twists)

dash of olive oil

3 tbsp sesame oil

3 cloves garlic, crushed

100 g carrots, peeled and cut into ribbons

200 g shredded young cabbage

5–6 tbsp dark soy sauce

2 tbsp toasted sesame seeds

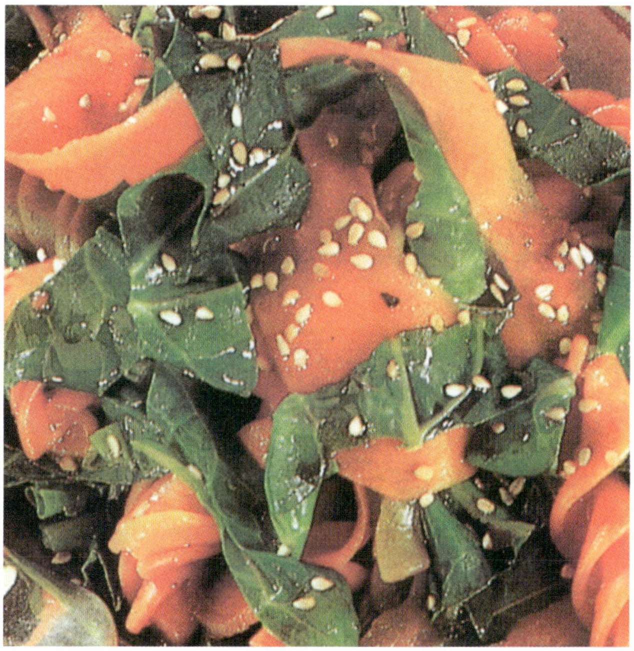

1. Bring a large saucepan of water to the boil, and add the fusilli with a dash of olive oil. Cook for about 10 minutes, stirring occasionally, until the pasta is tender. Drain thoroughly, and set aside.

2. Heat the sesame oil in a wok or large frying pan, and add the garlic. Stir-fry for 30 seconds, then add the carrot ribbons. Continue to cook for 3–4 minutes, then add the shredded cabbage. Cook for 2–3 minutes, stirring continuously.

3. Stir in the soy sauce, sesame seeds, and fusilli. Cook for a further 2 minutes, and serve immediately.

NUTRITIONAL VALUES

GREEN VEGETABLE RISOTTO

SERVES **4**

This dish makes an excellent accompaniment to meat or fish dishes, and can also be served as a vegetarian main meal.

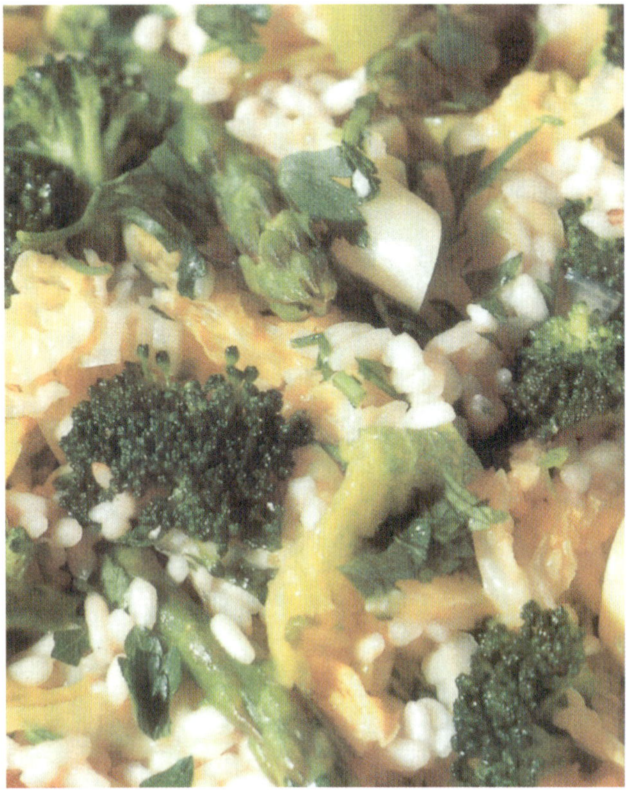

- 225 g small broccoli florets
- 100 g fine asparagus spears
- 225 g savoy cabbage, shredded
- 1 l vegetable stock
- 50 g garlic and herb butter
- 4 trimmed and shredded small leeks
- 400 g arborio rice
- salt substitute (see page 18) and freshly ground black pepper
- 4 tbsp chopped fresh parsley

1. Bring a saucepan of water to the boil and cook the broccoli for 3–4 minutes until just tender; cook the asparagus and cabbage for 1 minute until just tender. Drain the vegetables and set aside. Reserve the cooking water and use to make up the stock.
2. Pour the stock into a saucepan and bring to the boil. Reduce the heat to a gentle simmer.
3. Meanwhile, melt the garlic and herb butter in a large saucepan and gently fry the leeks for 2–3 minutes until softened but not browned. Stir in the rice and cook, stirring, for 2 minutes until the rice is well coated in the leek mixture.
4. Add a ladleful of stock and cook gently over a medium heat, stirring, until absorbed. Season well. Continue adding the stock until the risotto becomes thick, but not sticky, and the rice is tender. This will take about 25 minutes.
5. Stir in the cooked vegetables and chopped parsley, and heat through for 2–3 minutes until hot. Serve immediately.

NUTRITIONAL VALUES

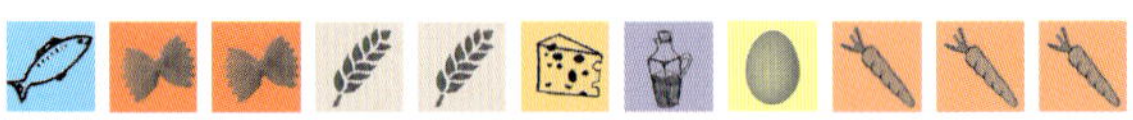

ITALIAN-STYLE STUFFED SQUASH

SERVES **4**

Butternut squash have a sweet, earthy flavour and a bright orange-yellow flesh. They make a stunning vegetable accompaniment because of their unusual long shape.

2 tbsp olive oil
1 medium red onion, peeled and chopped
1 tbsp lemon juice
2 cloves garlic, peeled and crushed
2 small butternut squash
black pepper
180 g cooked rice
2 large tomatoes, peeled, deseeded and chopped
40 g pitted black olives in brine, drained and chopped
1 small bunch basil, shredded
3 tbsp grated Parmesan cheese
basil leaves, to garnish

1 Presoak a large claypot as directed. Heat the oil in a small saucepan. Add the onion, lemon juice and garlic and fry gently for 3–4 minutes until just softened. Transfer to a mixing bowl to cool.

2 Meanwhile, cut the squash in half lengthways. Scoop out the fibre and seeds from the centre and season well. Mix the rice, tomatoes, olives and shredded basil into the cooked onion mixture. Season well and pile into the prepared squash.

3 Arrange in the claypot, cover, and place in a cold oven. Set the oven to 220°C/gas mark 7, and cook for 45 minutes. Remove the lid, sprinkle with the cheese, and cook for a further 15 minutes, until crisp and golden. Garnish with basil leaves to serve.

NUTRITIONAL VALUES

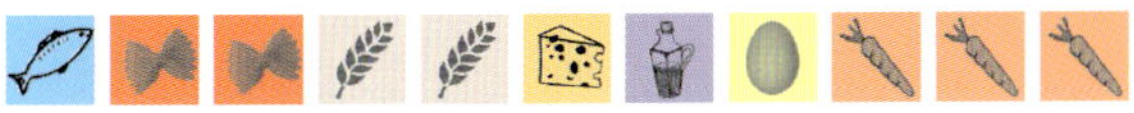

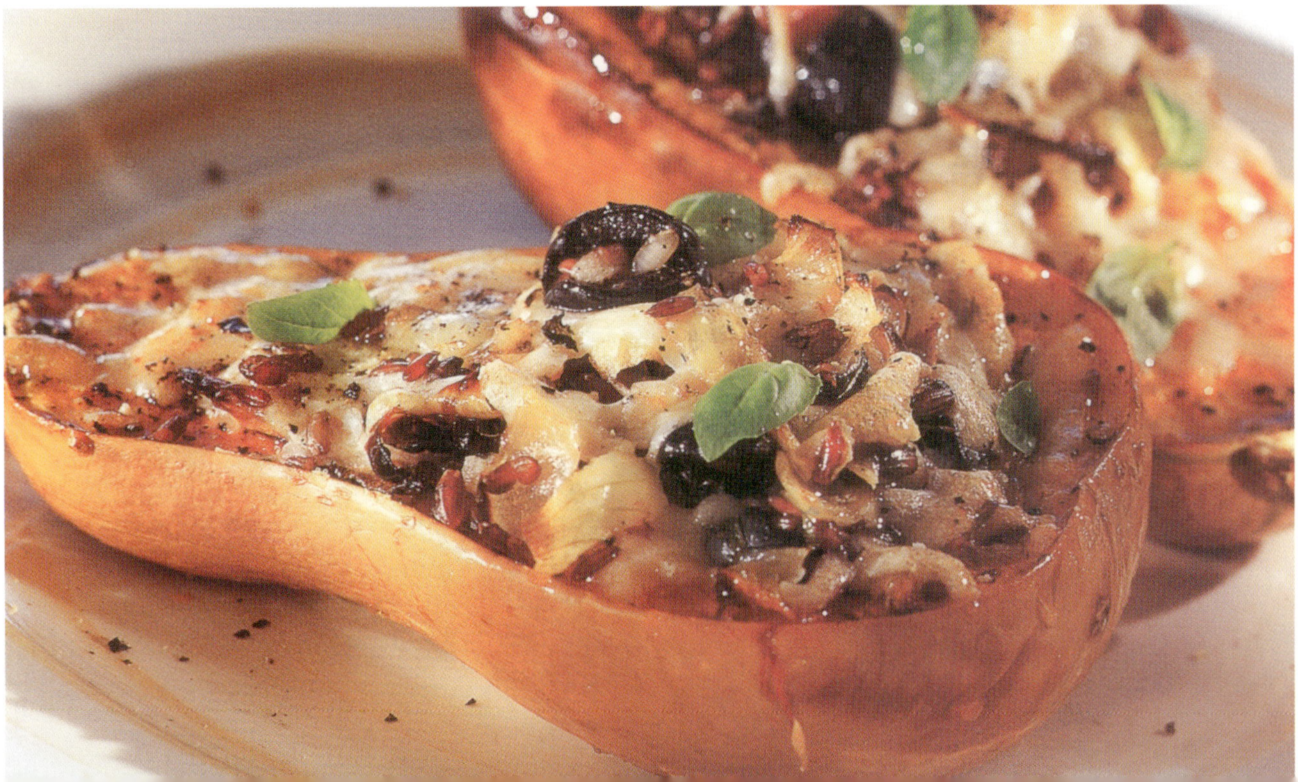

SQUASH, CUCUMBER AND BULGUR WHEAT SALAD

SERVES **8**

Tabbouleh, a mix of bulgur wheat and cucumber, with lots of chopped mint and parsley, is a traditional Middle Eastern salad which is very fashionable today.

125 g fine bulgur wheat
450 ml boiling water
225 g cucumber, finely diced
225 g diced and roasted winter squash, such as crown prince, butternut or kabocha
75 g chopped fresh parsley
3 tbsp chopped coriander
2 tomatoes, deseeded and chopped
2 spring onions, sliced
45 g toasted almonds, chopped
juice of 1 lemon
freshly ground black pepper
63 ml extra virgin olive oil

NUTRITIONAL VALUES

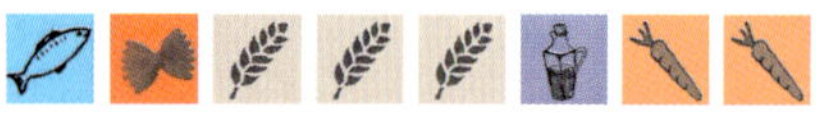

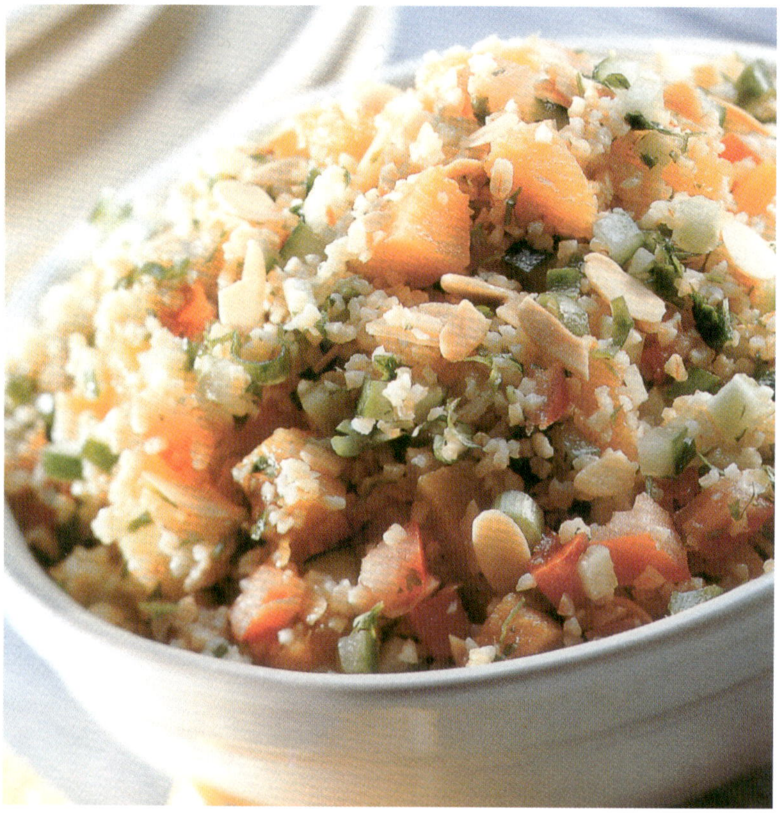

1 Soak the bulgur wheat in the boiling water and let stand for 30 minutes. Squeeze the grains dry in a dish towel, then turn them into a large salad bowl.

2 Add all the remaining ingredients, with plenty of seasoning to taste. Toss the salad well, then serve at room temperature.

SPICED COURGETTE AND ROASTED SQUASH SALAD

SERVES **6**

Seasoned with the exotic flavourings of Morocco, this salad makes an extremely useful addition to a buffet table as it is economical to make and very filling.

1 butternut squash (weighing about 1 kg)
freshly ground black pepper
extra virgin olive oil
180 g sliced courgettes
75 g pumpkin seeds, toasted if wished

FOR THE DRESSING

3 tbsp olive oil
2 tbsp white wine vinegar
1 green chilli, finely chopped
1 tsp chilli sauce
pinch of ground cumin
pinch of ground cinnamon
2 tbsp chopped fresh coriander

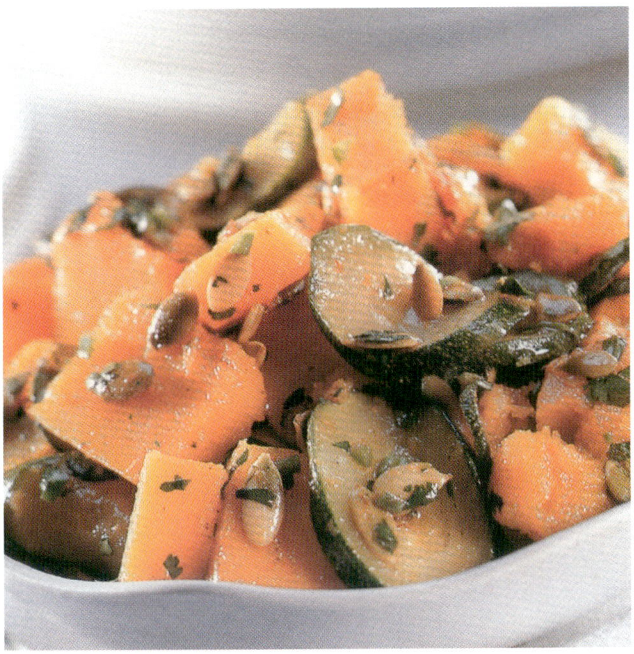

1 Preheat the oven to 220°C/gas mark 7 oven. Cut the squash in half and scoop out the seeds, then arrange the halves in a small roasting pan. Season lightly, drizzle with olive oil, then roast for 30–5 minutes, or until tender.

2 Fry the courgettes in 4 tablespoons oil until just starting to brown, but still quite firm. Scoop them out of the pan into a large salad bowl.

3 Blend the dressing ingredients with the oil left in the pan, and season to taste.

4 Scoop the flesh out of the skins of the squash and chop roughly. Add the squash to the courgettes, with the pumpkin seeds, and toss well, then pour the dressing over.

NUTRITIONAL VALUES

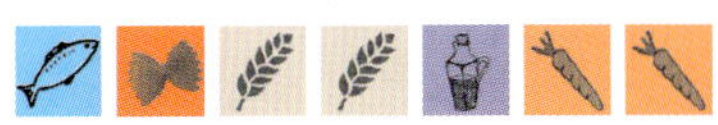

EGGS FLORENTINE

SERVES **8**

This is a popular breakfast, brunch or supper dish.

8 medium eggs
450 g fresh spinach, tough stalks discarded and well washed
4 tbsp olive oil
1 small onion, finely chopped
1–2 garlic cloves, crushed
40 g plain flour
250 ml skimmed milk
1 tsp Dijon mustard
freshly ground black pepper
63 g Gruyère cheese, grated
warm, crusty bread, to serve

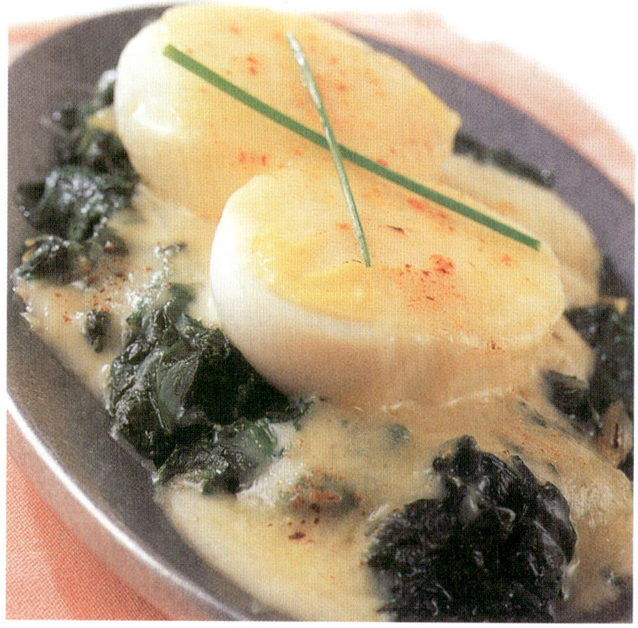

1 Place the eggs in a heavy saucepan, cover with cold water, and bring to the boil. Boil gently for 10 minutes, then plunge into cold water. Leave until cool. Peel and cut in half.

2 Meanwhile, place the spinach with water just clinging to the leaves in a heavy saucepan. Cover with a lid and cook for 3–4 minutes. Drain and chop finely. Heat 1 tablespoon of the olive oil in a small frying pan. Gently sauté the onion and garlic for 5 minutes or until softened. Stir in the spinach, then place in the base of an ovenproof gratin dish. Place the boiled egg halves on top.

3 Heat the remaining olive oil in a small heavy saucepan. Stir in the flour and cook for 2 minutes. Remove from the heat and gradually stir in the milk. Return to the heat and cook, stirring, until the mixture thickens and coats the back of a wooden spoon. Remove from the heat and stir in the mustard, seasoning, and half the cheese.

4 To serve, preheat the grill to medium. Pour the sauce over the eggs. Sprinkle with the remaining cheese and place under the grill for 8–10 minutes, or until golden brown and bubbly. Serve immediately with warm, crusty bread.

NUTRITIONAL VALUES

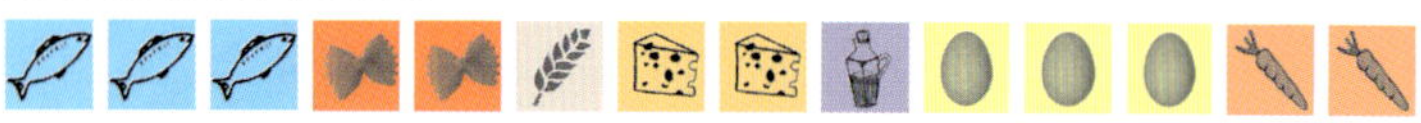

SQUID WITH BEETROOT

SERVES **4**

Squid is a popular ingredient in the Mediterranean, and after tasting this dish you will understand why.

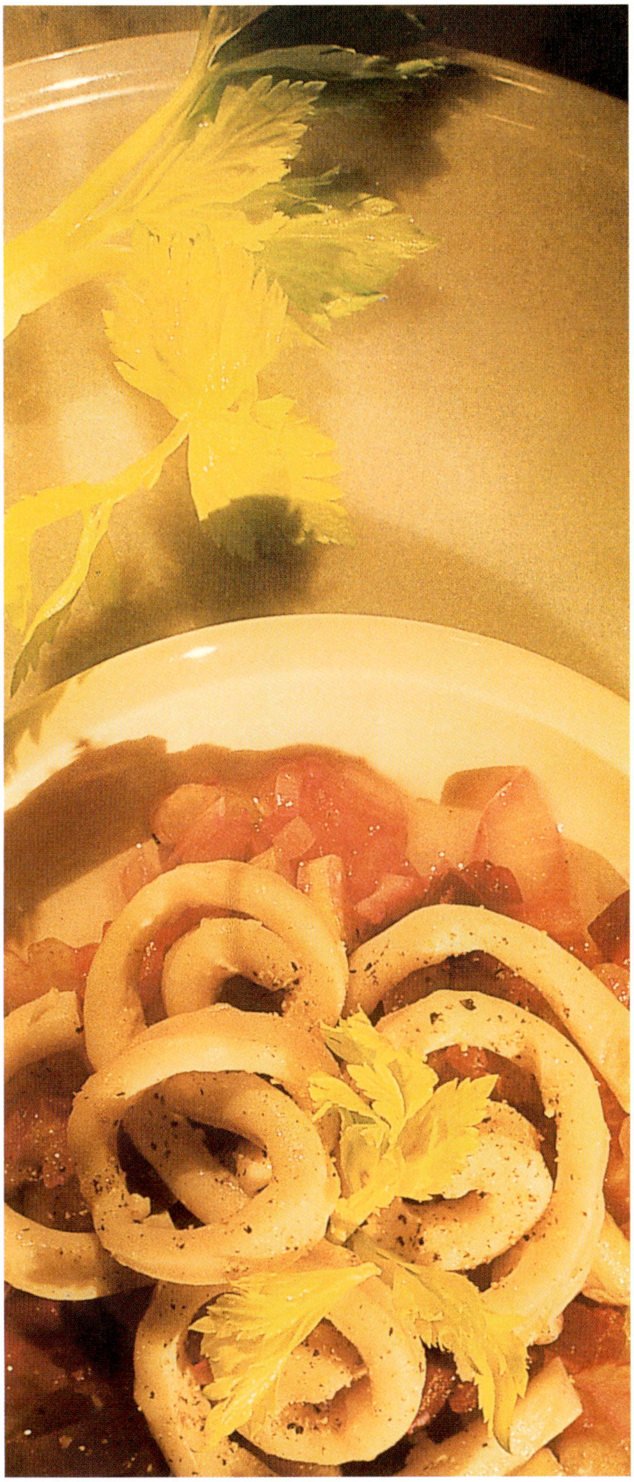

450 g small squid
1 tbsp olive oil
1 small onion, chopped
1 clove garlic, crushed
1 celery stick, finely chopped
2 cooked beetroot, chopped
3 tbsp dry white wine
1 tbsp tomato purée
fresh ground black pepper
celery tips

1 First clean the squid. Remove the eyes, mouth, ink sac, 'nib' and outer membrane. Wash the squid well, then slice the body and tentacles.

2 Put the olive oil in a microwave-safe pot and cook on full for 30 seconds. Stir in the onion and garlic and cook on full for 2 minutes.

3 Add the celery, beetroot and squid. Mix the white wine and tomato purée and pour over the squid. Cover and cook for 8 minutes, or until the squid is tender.

4 Season with pepper and serve garnished with celery tips.

NUTRITIONAL VALUES

GARLIC NEW POTATOES

SERVES **4**

New potatoes are just young potatoes, of any variety. Choose firm, well-shaped and blemish-free potatoes of roughly equal size, so that they all cook in the same amount of time.

450 g new potatoes, lightly scrubbed

2 tbsp olive oil

2 garlic cloves, peeled and crushed

1 tbsp fresh basil, chopped

FOR THE SAUCE

1 small onion, quartered, and thinly sliced

1 tsp paprika

pinch of cayenne pepper

1 tsp fennel seeds

300 ml passata

300 ml vegetable stock

2 tbsp fresh basil, chopped

fresh basil, to garnish

1. Line a steamer tier with foil, making an edge to form a dish. Put the potatoes, oil, garlic and basil in the foil.

2. Place the sauce ingredients in the base of the steamer and bring to the boil. Cook the potatoes, covered, over the sauce for 45 minutes until the potatoes are tender. Garnish with basil, and serve with the sauce.

NUTRITIONAL VALUES

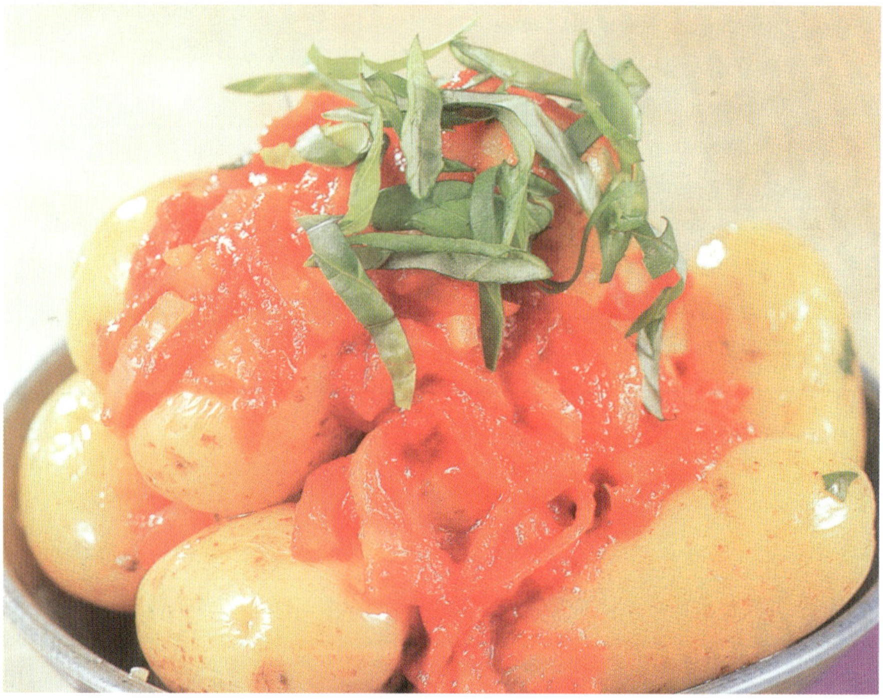

SHREDDED CHICKEN SALAD WITH GARLIC-ROASTED PEPPERS AND CHILLIES

SERVES **4**

All the components of this salad can be prepared in advance so, if you have some cooked chicken left over from a roast dinner, this is the perfect way of using it up. However, it is so delicious that it is well worth poaching some chicken just for this salad.

3 tbsp olive oil
4 garlic cloves
1 large red pepper, quartered, and deseeded
1 large yellow or orange pepper, quartered, and deseeded
3 large red chillies, deseeded
600 ml chicken or vegetable stock
freshly ground black pepper
2 large skinless, boneless, chicken breasts
60 g rocket or other green salad leaves

DRESSING

4 tbsp natural yoghurt
3 tbsp olive oil
1 tbsp white wine vinegar
1 garlic clove, crushed
1 tbsp finely chopped fresh mint
salt substitute (see page 18) and freshly ground black pepper

NUTRITIONAL VALUES

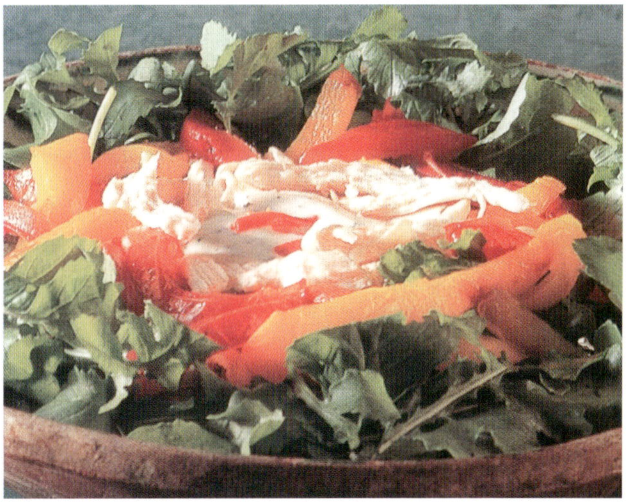

1 Preheat the oven to 190°C/gas mark 5. Put the olive oil in a shallow roasting tin and heat it gently in the pre-heated oven or on the hob. Bruise the garlic cloves with the back of a spoon and add them to the oil. Add the pieces of pepper and whole chillies to the oil and mix well. Roast in the oven for 35 minutes. Once roasted, allow the peppers to cool and discard the garlic.

2 Meanwhile, pour the stock into an ovenproof dish and season with salt substitute and freshly ground black pepper. Add the chicken breasts and cover with foil. Poach in the oven for 20 minutes. Remove the breasts from the stock and leave them to cool. Once cooled, shred each breast.

3 To make the dressing, combine all the ingredients in a screw-topped jar and shake well. Set aside.

4 Place the salad leaves in a large bowl. Once the roasted vegetables have cooled, slice the peppers into strips about 1 cm thick and thinly slice the chillies. Toss together the peppers, chillies and shredded chicken and arrange on top of the salad leaves. Shake the dressing again and then pour it over the salad and serve at once.

STUFFED CABBAGE LEAVES

SERVES **4**

What better way to impress your dinner guests than with these stuffed cabbage leaves? They are high in flavour and antioxidants.

1 large green cabbage, or 450 g spinach
1 tsp paprika
freshly ground black pepper
$^1/_2$ tbsp parsley, chopped
500 g lamb, minced
4 tbsp olive oil
1 onion, finely chopped
1 tsp garlic, crushed
1 red chilli, deseeded and chopped
1 tsp tomato purée
250 ml tomato juice
1 tsp soy sauce
300 ml chicken broth
75 g mushrooms, finely chopped
56 g salted peanuts, crushed

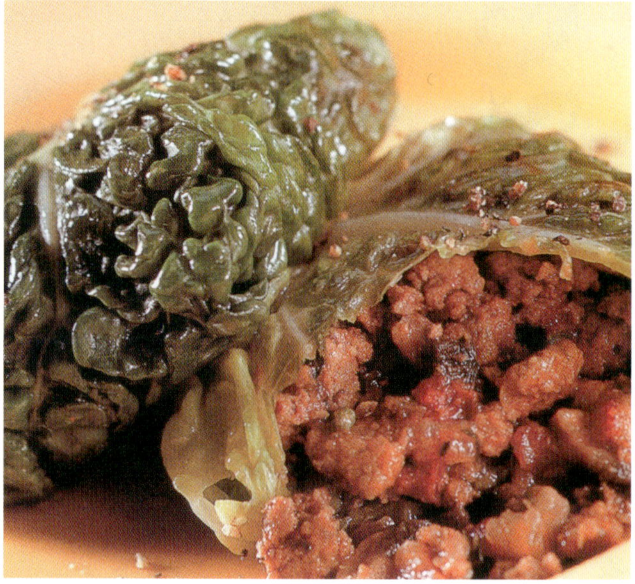

NUTRITIONAL VALUES

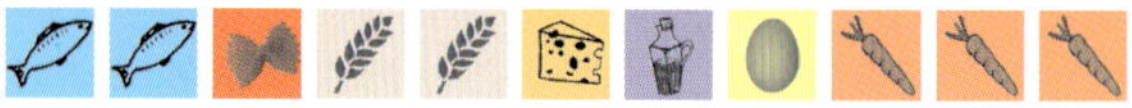

1 Remove the dirty outer leaves from the cabbage. Carefully pick off the large whole leaves and cut out the thick part of the stalk. Put the leaves in a pot of boiling water to soften. Simmer for 5 minutes.

2 Remove the leaves and plunge into cold water. When cold, carefully lay out the leaves on a clean tea towel or kitchen towel, and pat dry with another tea towel placed on top. Arrange with the inside of the leaves facing towards you.

TO PREPARE THE FILLING

3 In a large bowl, work the paprika, pepper and parsley into the minced lamb.

4 Heat the olive oil in a pan. Add the onion and cook gently until softened. Add the lamb, garlic, chilli and tomato purée. Pour in the tomato juice, soy sauce, and broth, and stir. Add the mushrooms and peanuts.

5 Simmer for 30 minutes, stirring occasionally. Remove from the heat and cool. Check the seasoning. If the mixture is still runny, add a small amount of flour.

6 When cold, spoon small amounts of the mixture into the centre of the cabbage leaves, folding the outside edges over and placing the folded side, base down, in an oiled baking tray.

Note: If your leaves are a little ragged or small, use two leaves to wrap around the lamb mixture.

7 When all the cabbage parcels are in the baking pan, pour in enough chicken broth to half-cover them. Cover the tray with foil. Pierce with a fork to allow the steam to escape and poach in the oven for 20 minutes, at 200°C/gas mark 6.

8 Remove carefully with a large spoon and moisten with a little of the poaching liquor.

STARTERS

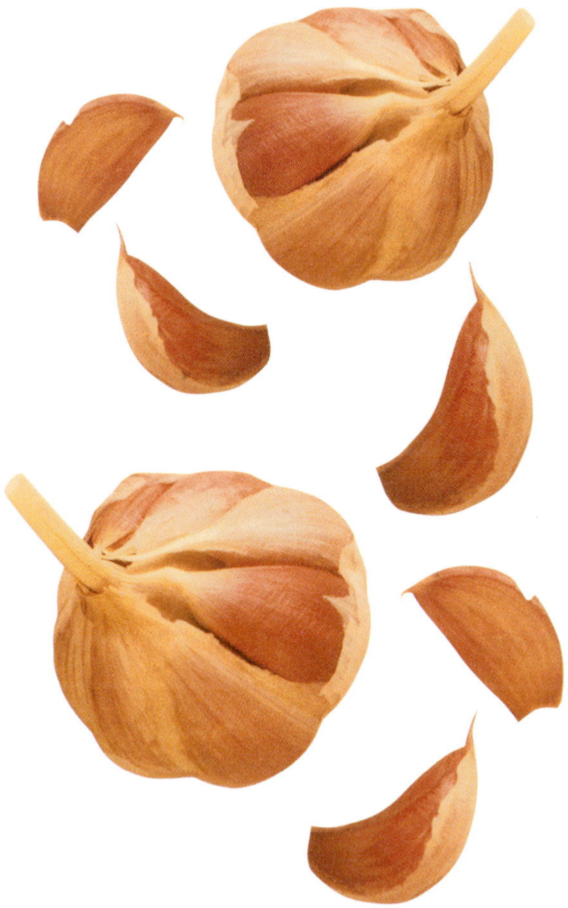

QUICK ASIAN GREENS SOUP

SERVES **1**

This is an easy-to-prepare lunch that can be made when you are pressed for time. It is light and goes well with a bowl of steamed rice or some hot crusty bread.

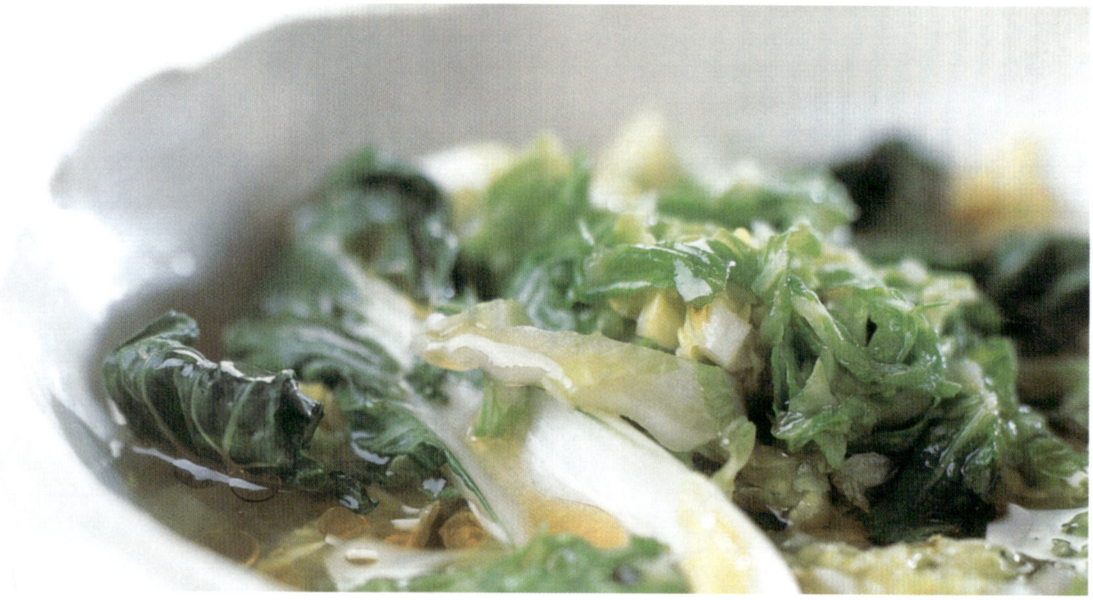

400 g carton chicken stock
4 napa cabbage leaves, julienned
1 stalk baby bok choy or Shanghai bok choy
white pepper

1. In a pan, bring the chicken stock to the boil.
2. Add the napa cabbage, bring to the boil then simmer for 3–4 minutes.
3. Add the bok choy and simmer for a further 2–3 minutes or until tender.
4. Remove from the heat, stir in the sesame oil and a dash of pepper. Serve piping hot.

NUTRITIONAL VALUES

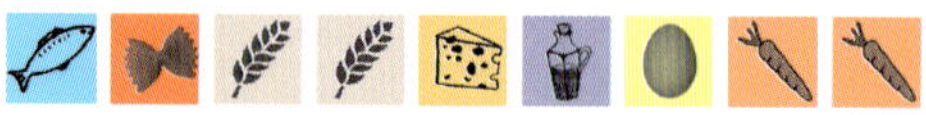

WHITE RADISH SOUP

SERVES **4-6**

This soup is warming, soothing and comes from Korea, where it is usually served for breakfast.

16 dried Chinese mushrooms, soaked in hot water for 30 minutes
2 litres chicken stock
450 g diced white radish
275 g mung bean sprouts
1 tsp soy sauce
$^1/_2$ tsp sugar
freshly ground black pepper

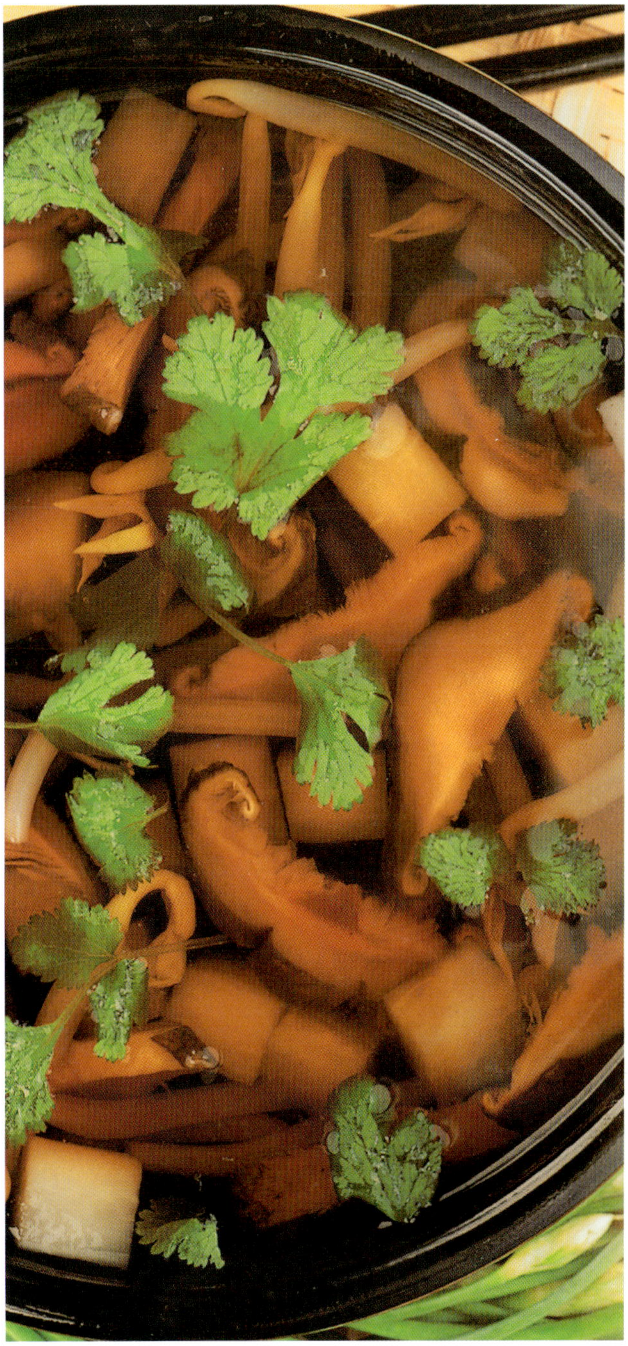

1 Remove the mushrooms from the soaking water. Drain and reserve the water.

2 Remove and discard the stalks from the mushrooms. Thinly slice the caps and put into a large pan with the stock.

3 Bring to the boil and add the white radish. Cover the pan and simmer slowly for about 10 minutes until the white radish is tender.

4 Add the bean sprouts, return to the boil. Cover again and simmer for 3–4 minutes more. Add the soy sauce, sugar and pepper.

NUTRITIONAL VALUES

TLALPENO-STYLE SOUP

SERVES **4**

Sometimes this Mexican soup is made with a chicken stock; sometimes with vegetable stock. Usually it contains some kind of chilli pepper, though which sort of pepper varies widely. Some versions usually contain little or no garlic; Mexican versions may contain a whole head. This is a simple, authentic version, for four modest servings.

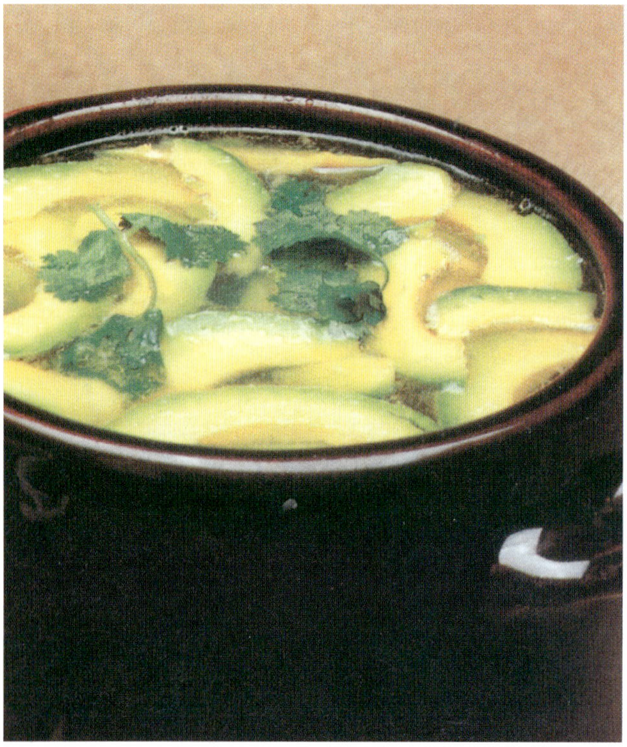

100 g chicken (white meat)
900 ml chicken stock
1 or 2 dried red chillies
1–5 cloves garlic
3 tbsp water
1 avocado
coriander (about half a handful) to garnish

1 Slice the chicken into julienne strips. If the chicken is not cooked, bring the chicken stock to a boil; simmer the meat until it is cooked (less than 5 minutes). Otherwise, bring the stock and chicken to a simmering boil. Doubling the amount of chicken will not do any harm.

2 Deseed the chillies; tear into pieces; grind in a pestle and mortar with the garlic and 3 tablespoons of water. Strain into the stock. Stir, then simmer for a couple of minutes.

3 Peel the avocado and slice into strips. Separate the slices carefully before dropping them into the soup, or they will stick together. They will sink for a few moments, then float to the surface. When they do, the soup is ready. Chop some coriander and float it on the surface for a garnish.

NUTRITIONAL VALUES

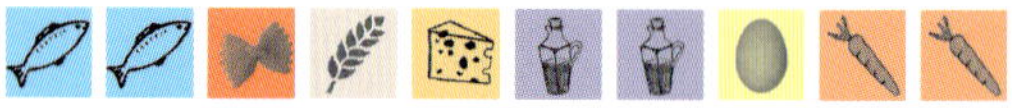

LEMON AND PARSLEY SOUP

SERVES **4**

This mouth-watering combination of lemon and chicken flavours is the perfect start to any meal.

2 tbsp olive oil
4 bunches flatleaf parsley, stalks removed (about 6 oz leaves)
1 tsp ground coriander
2 garlic cloves, crushed and peeled
750 ml rich chicken stock
4 tbsp freshly squeezed lemon juice
1 tbsp grated lemon zest
500 ml plain low-fat yoghurt
freshly ground black pepper
parsley leaves to garnish (optional)
lemon zest to garnish (optional)

1 Heat the olive oil in a large non-reactive saucepan over medium heat. Add the parsley leaves and cook, tossing frequently, until the leaves are completely wilted and coated with oil (about 3–5 minutes). Add the coriander and garlic and sauté for 2 minutes longer. Add the stock, lemon juice and lemon zest. Bring the mixture to the boil, then lower the heat and simmer for 10 minutes.

2 Remove the soup from the heat and purée in batches. Wipe out the pan and return the soup to it. Add the yoghurt and mix thoroughly.

3 If you are serving the soup cold, allow it to cool, then cover and refrigerate it until it is well chilled.

4 If you are serving it hot, heat the soup through, but do not let it boil.

5 When serving, season with pepper to taste and garnish with parsley and lemon zest, if desired.

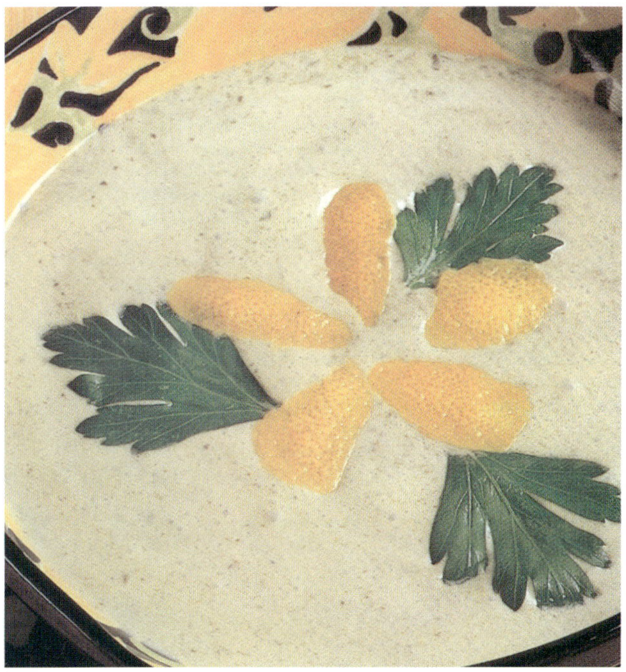

NUTRITIONAL VALUES

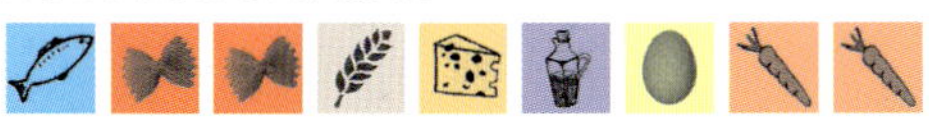

BEETROOT BORTSCH

SERVES **6**

There are many versions of bortsch; the only ingredient which does not vary is the beetroot! This soup is made all over Eastern Europe and served hot or cold. It can be made with beef or without, with vegetables or without, and served chunky or smooth. This elegant ruby-red purée is most delicious served with a swirl of low-fat sour cream, snipped chives and dill.

750 g small beetroot with tops
1 onion, chopped
900 ml beef, chicken or vegetable stock, or water
1 tsp salt
freshly ground black pepper
3 tbsp fresh lemon juice
2 tbsp light brown sugar, or to taste
low-fat yogurt for serving
snipped fresh chives and dill for garnish

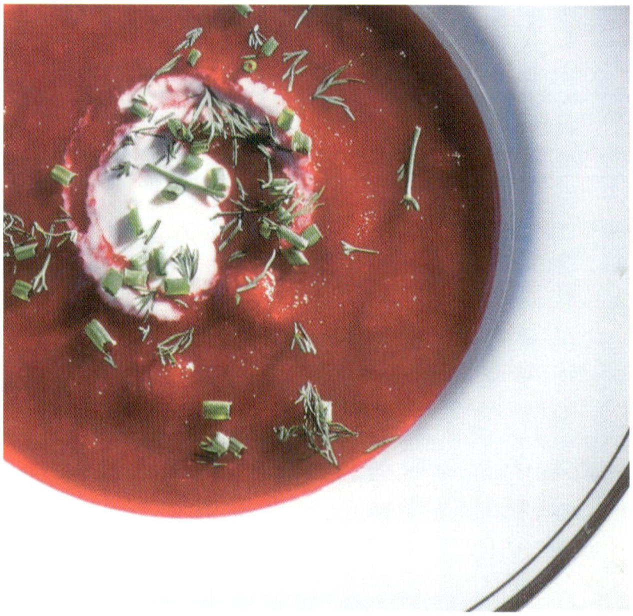

1. Cut the tops from the beetroot, leaving 5 to 7.5 cm of stalk attached. Scrub the beetroot thoroughly under cold running water, being sure to remove all grit and sand. If the tops are young and tender they may be added, well washed.

2. In a large saucepan, over medium heat, place the beetroot and chopped onion and cover with stock or water. Bring to the boil, then simmer, partially covered, until the beetroot is tender, 20–30 minutes. Carefully strain the liquid through a sieve into a large heatproof bowl; rinse saucepan.

3. Remove the beetroot and peel off skin. Quarter the beetroot and add to a food processor fitted with metal blade. Add the onions (and tops if using) from the sieve to the beetroot; process until finely puréed.

4. Return the beetroot and onion purée to the washed saucepan and add the reserved cooking liquid, being careful not to add any sand or grit which may have settled on the bottom.

5. Over medium heat, bring the soup to the boil. Season with pepper and lemon. Simmer for 5 minutes and serve hot with a swirl of low-fat yoghurt. Sprinkle with fresh chives and dill. Alternatively, cool and chill to serve cold.

NUTRITIONAL VALUES

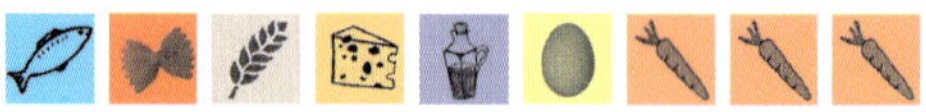

SPINACH AND YOGHURT SOUP

SERVES **6**

Popular in Egypt, Jordan and Lebanon, this soup is more usually made with beetroot greens, which impart a characteristic, slightly sour flavour. When the more easily obtainable spinach is used, as in this recipe, a touch of light white wine vinegar will help to approximate the taste.

1 garlic clove, minced
475 ml Greek-style yoghurt
large pinch turmeric
3 tbsp olive oil
1 large onion, finely chopped
450 g spinach leaves, washed thoroughly and shredded
2 small leeks, finely chopped
100 g long-grain rice
1 l vegetable stock
3 tbsp white wine vinegar (champagne vinegar, if available)
freshly ground black pepper

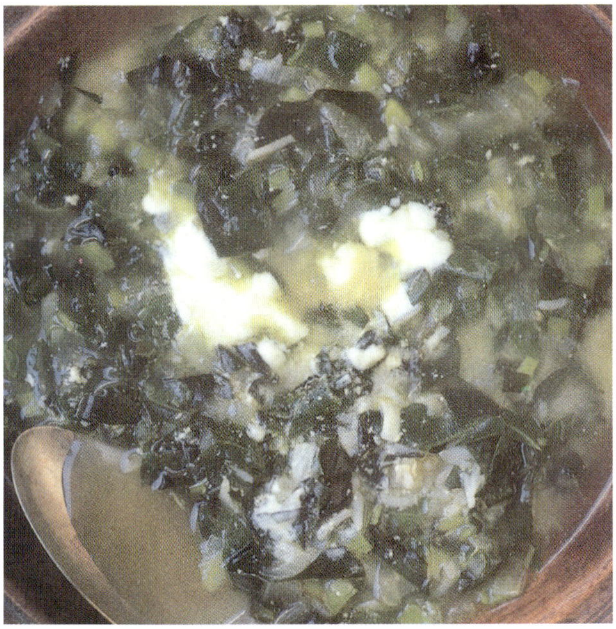

1 In a bowl, whisk together the garlic, yoghurt and turmeric. Set aside to let the flavours mingle.

2 Heat the olive oil in a large casserole and stir in the onion. Sauté until lightly coloured and softened, then stir in the spinach, leeks, and rice. When the spinach has wilted and the rice is coated, pour in the vegetable stock and the vinegar. Season to taste. Bring to the boil, then reduce the heat, cover and simmer for about 15–20 minutes, until the rice is tender.

3 Just before serving, take the soup off the heat. Whisk in the yoghurt mixture, and then ladle immediately into bowls.

NUTRITIONAL VALUES

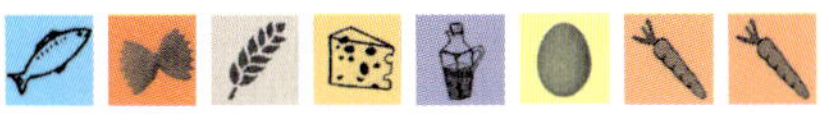

PARSNIP AND APPLE SOUP

SERVES **4–6**

Curried parsnip is one of the new generation of classic soups. Add a cooking apple to the mixture if you like – its sharpness gives a real punch to the flavour of the soup.

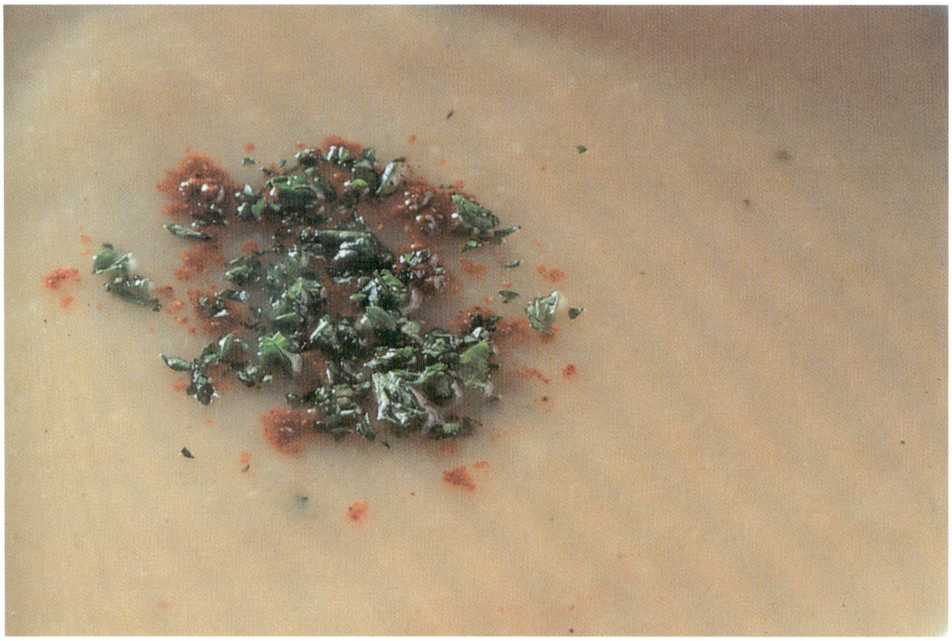

1 onion, chopped
1 tbsp sunflower oil
1 tsp mild curry powder
450 g parsnips, chopped
1 cooking apple, peeled, cored and sliced
1.2 litres well-flavoured vegetable stock
freshly ground black pepper
juice of $^1/_2$ lemon
chopped fresh parsley or coriander, to garnish

1 Cook the onion in the oil for 4–5 minutes until soft, then stir in the curry powder with the parsnips. Cook for a further 2–3 minutes before adding the apple and stock. Bring to the boil, then simmer for 30 minutes or until the parsnip is soft.

2 Allow the soup to cool slightly, then purée until smooth in a blender or food processor. Rinse the pan and return the soup to it, adding sufficient water to thin the soup if necessary. Reheat gently, then season to taste with pepper. Add the lemon juice just before serving and garnish with parsley or coriander.

NUTRITIONAL VALUES

TUSCAN WHITE BEAN AND KALE SOUP

SERVES **6**

This soup is perfect for a fireside supper on a winter's evening. It is high in fibre and antioxidants and can be served with warm wholegrain bread or garlic bread.

225 g dried borlotti beans, soaked overnight in cold water to cover generously
1 tbsp olive oil
100 g pancetta or smoked lean bacon, chopped
1 onion, finely chopped
1 shallot, finely chopped
1 carrot, finely chopped
1–2 garlic cloves, minced
4 tomatoes, peeled, deseeded and chopped, or 438 ml canned chopped tomatoes
1.2 litres water
bouquet garni (thyme and marjoram sprigs, parsley stems and bay leaf)
125 g curly kale leaves, finely chopped
freshly grated or shaved Parmesan cheese, for serving (optional)

1 Drain the beans, put into a saucepan with cold water to cover and set over high heat. Bring to the boil, and boil for 10 minutes. Drain and add fresh cold water to cover. Bring to the boil again, drain and rinse well.

2 Heat the oil in a large heavy saucepan over medium-high heat and add the pancetta or bacon. Cook until lightly browned, stirring frequently. Remove with a slotted spoon to drain on paper towels and pour off all but 1 tablespoon of the fat. Reduce the heat to low, add the onion, shallot, carrot and garlic, and cook for 3–4 minutes until slightly softened. Add the beans, tomatoes, water, bouquet garni, and pancetta or bacon, and simmer until the beans are tender, 1–2 hours. Season to taste with pepper.

3 Stir in the kale and continue cooking for 15–20 minutes, or until it is tender. Adjust the seasoning and ladle the soup into warm bowls. Serve sprinkled with Parmesan cheese, if you wish.

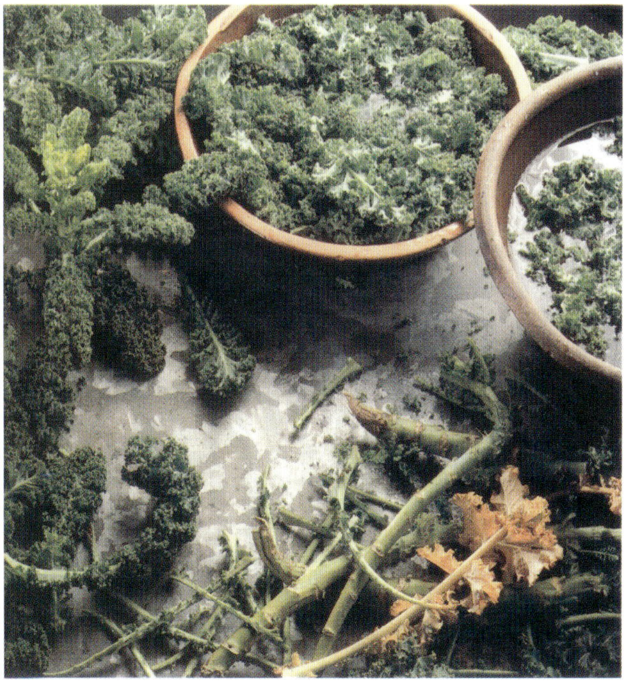

NUTRITIONAL VALUES

ROASTED GARLIC SOUP

SERVES **4**

This soup has a mellow, almost smoky, garlic flavour that makes it immensely satisfying yet very light. A strong well-flavoured stock is essential and it should be relatively clear, to see the croûtons. It is inspired by the Mediterranean peasant soups found in France, Italy, Spain and Portugal.

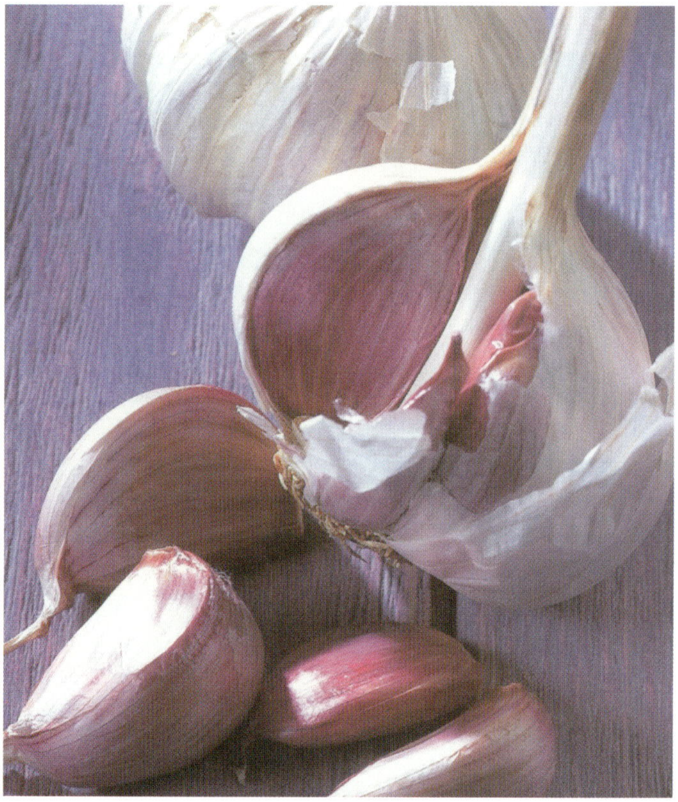

1 large head large-clove garlic, about 100 g
1 litre chicken or beef stock
2–3 slices wholemeal bread, crusts trimmed
finely chopped fresh parsley, for garnishing

NUTRITIONAL VALUES

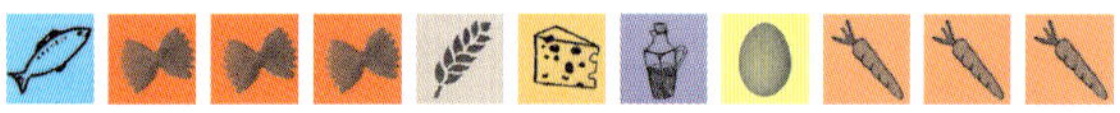

1 Preheat the oven to 200°C/gas mark 6. Wrap the garlic, whole, in foil and bake for about 40 minutes until very soft.

2 Bring the stock just to the boil over medium heat. Remove and set aside 3 cloves of the garlic, put the rest of the head into the stock and press with a wooden spoon to crush it lightly. Reduce the heat to low and simmer gently, partially covered, for 30 minutes, or until the stock has taken on the flavour of the garlic.

3 Cut the bread into 12 squares or diamond shapes about 3 cm on each side. Place on a baking sheet and toast the bread lightly. Squeeze out the garlic from the reserved garlic cloves and spread on the croûtons.

4 Place the croûtons in the bottom of warm soup plates. Strain the soup to remove the garlic and ladle it over the croûtons, dividing evenly among the soup plates. Sprinkle with parsley and serve.

FENNEL AND WALNUT SOUP

SERVES **4–6**

An aniseed-flavoured soup with the fine texture of chopped walnuts. This sophisticated soup makes an excellent dinner party appetizer. Reserve any celery leaves and fennel fronds for garnish.

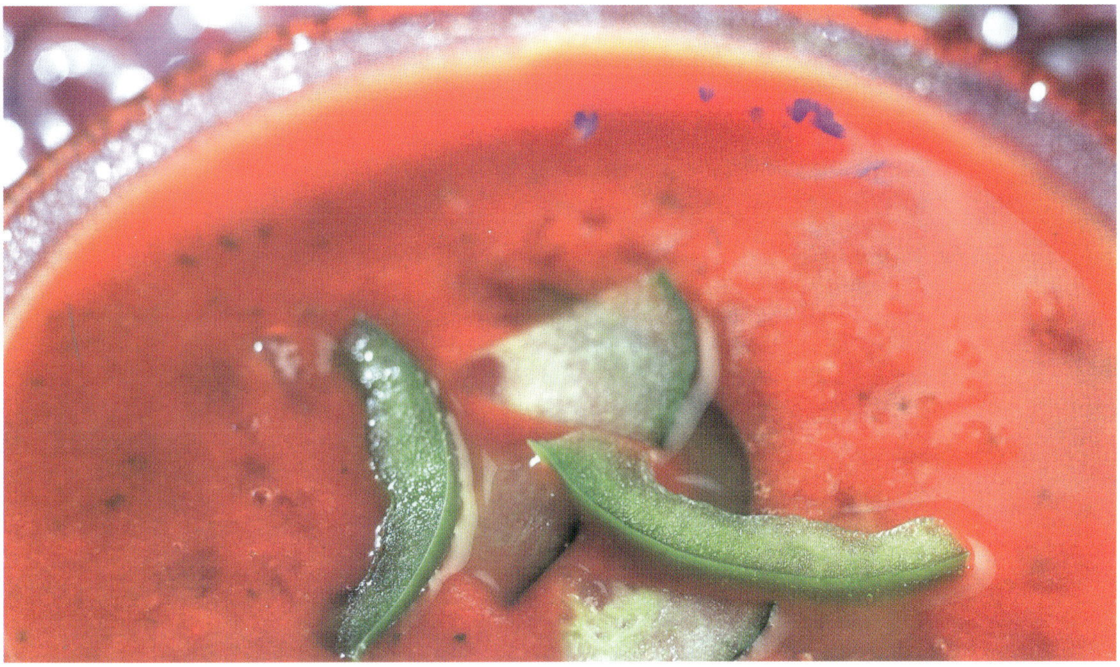

1 onion, finely chopped
1 head fennel, trimmed and sliced
3 sticks celery, trimmed and sliced
2 tbsp olive oil
1 plump clove garlic, finely sliced
2 bay leaves
1.35 litres vegetable stock
freshly ground black pepper
150 ml low-fat plain yoghurt
50 g walnuts, chopped finely
freshly chopped parsley mixed with fennel fronds and celery leaves to garnish

1 Cook the prepared vegetables slowly in the oil until soft but not browned. Add the garlic, bay leaves and stock and bring the soup to the boil. Cover the pan and simmer for 30–40 minutes, until the vegetables are tender.

2 Cool the soup slightly and remove the bay leaves. Then purée until smooth in a blender or food processor. Rinse the pan and return the soup to it. Reheat gently and season to taste with pepper, then stir in the low-fat yoghurt. Add the walnuts just before serving and garnish with any reserved chopped fennel fronds and celery leaves mixed with parsley.

NUTRITIONAL VALUES

BUTTERNUT AND ORANGE SOUP

SERVES **4–6**

This soup has a wonderful combination of flavours and is a good source of fibre. Do not boil the soup after adding the orange juice or the flavour will become slightly tainted.

1 onion, chopped
2 tbsp olive oil
1–2 butternut squash, weighing about 900 g, peeled and diced
grated rind and juice of 2 oranges
1.5 litres well-flavoured vegetable stock
freshly ground black pepper
2 bay leaves
freshly grated nutmeg
2 tbsp freshly chopped parsley

NUTRITIONAL VALUES

1 Cook the onion in the oil until softened but not browned, then add the prepared squash and cook slowly for 5 minutes, stirring occasionally. Stir in the grated orange rind, then add the broth, bay leaves and seasonings. Bring the soup to the boil then cover and simmer for 40 minutes, until the squash is tender and cooked through.

2 Allow the soup to cool slightly, remove the bay leaves, then purée in a blender or food processor until smooth. Rinse the pan and return the soup to it, adding the orange juice. Reheat the soup slowly – do not let it boil – then season to taste. Add the freshly chopped parsley just before serving.

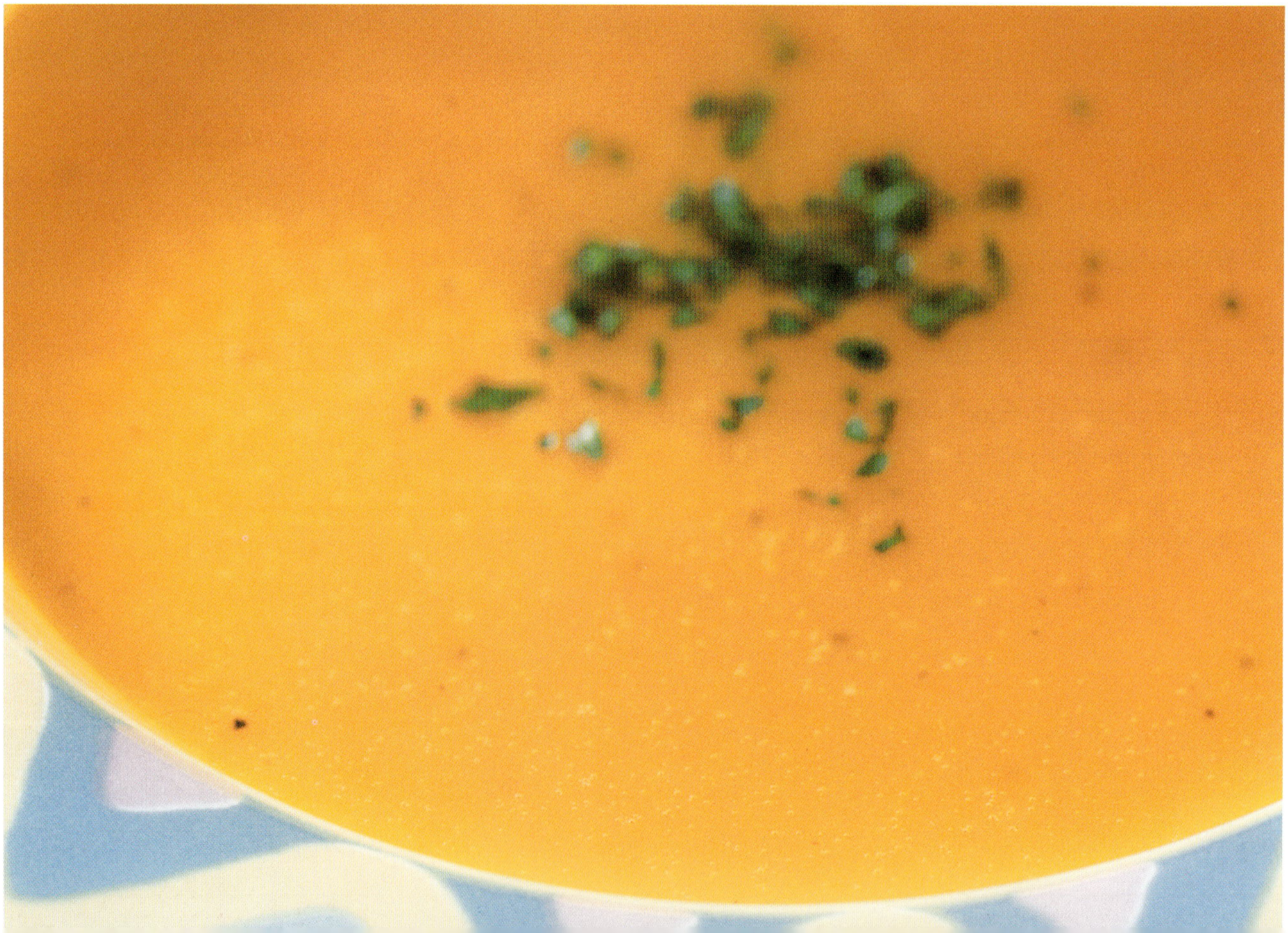

MINESTRA ALLA BOSCA

SERVES **4–6**

If you prefer to use something else other than turkey, this soup can be prepared with any sort of gamey meat, such as pheasant or wild rabbit.

275 g dark turkey meat, cut into bite-sized pieces
1 onion, chopped
1/2 carrot, chopped
1 bay leaf
3 tbsp extra virgin olive oil
1 tbsp flour
175 g wild rice
2 potatoes, peeled and diced
1.2 litres chicken, game or vegetable stock
25 g dried mushrooms, such as porcini
225 g common cultivated mushrooms, thinly sliced
4 tbsp dry sherry, Madeira or Marsala
freshly ground black pepper, to taste

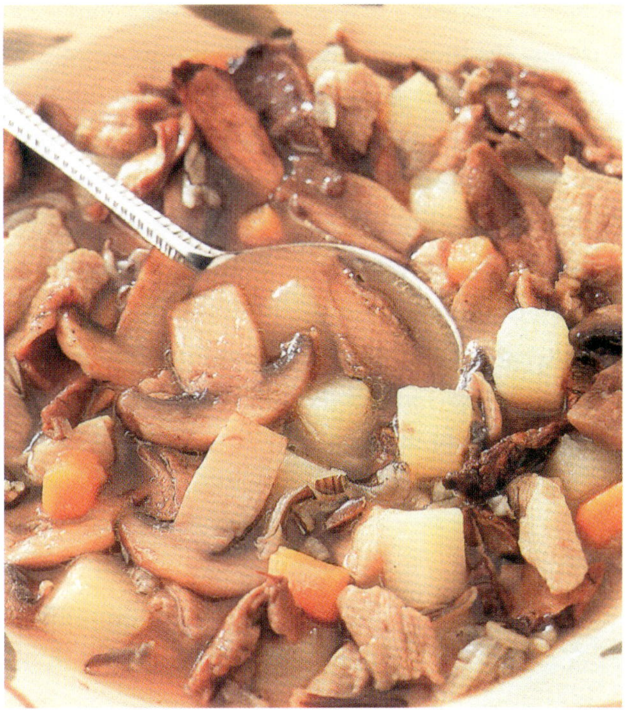

1 Sauté the turkey with the onion, carrot and bay leaf in 1 tablespoon of the olive oil until the onion is softened and the turkey is lightly browned. Sprinkle in the flour and stir well to cook the flour through.

2 Add the wild rice, potatoes and stock, and bring to the boil. Reduce the heat to a simmer and cook over low heat until the rice is nearly tender, about 45 minutes.

3 Meanwhile, rehydrate the mushrooms by pouring 225 ml hot, but not boiling, water over the mushrooms in a heatproof bowl. Cover and leave for about 30 minutes, then remove the mushrooms from the liquid and squeeze well over the bowl. Strain the soaking liquid and set aside.

4 Sauté the sliced fresh mushrooms in the remaining olive oil, then add the rehydrated mushrooms, and cook together for a few minutes until the fresh mushrooms are lightly browned.

5 Add the mushrooms to the soup mixture, along with the strained mushroom liquid. Pour in the sherry, Madeira or Marsala, and season to taste. Serve immediately.

NUTRITIONAL VALUES

ROAST CROWN PRINCE SQUASH AND PISTACHIO PÂTÉ

SERVES **6**

This really is a favourite recipe for squash. You won't miss meat, liver or fish in this thick pâté because the flavour and texture of the squash is wonderful. And it's so easy to make!

675 g crown prince squash, deseeded
salt substitute (see page 18) and freshly ground black pepper
olive oil
250 g low-fat cream cheese
1–2 garlic cloves, crushed
1 hot red chilli, deseeded and finely chopped
50 g pistachios, chopped

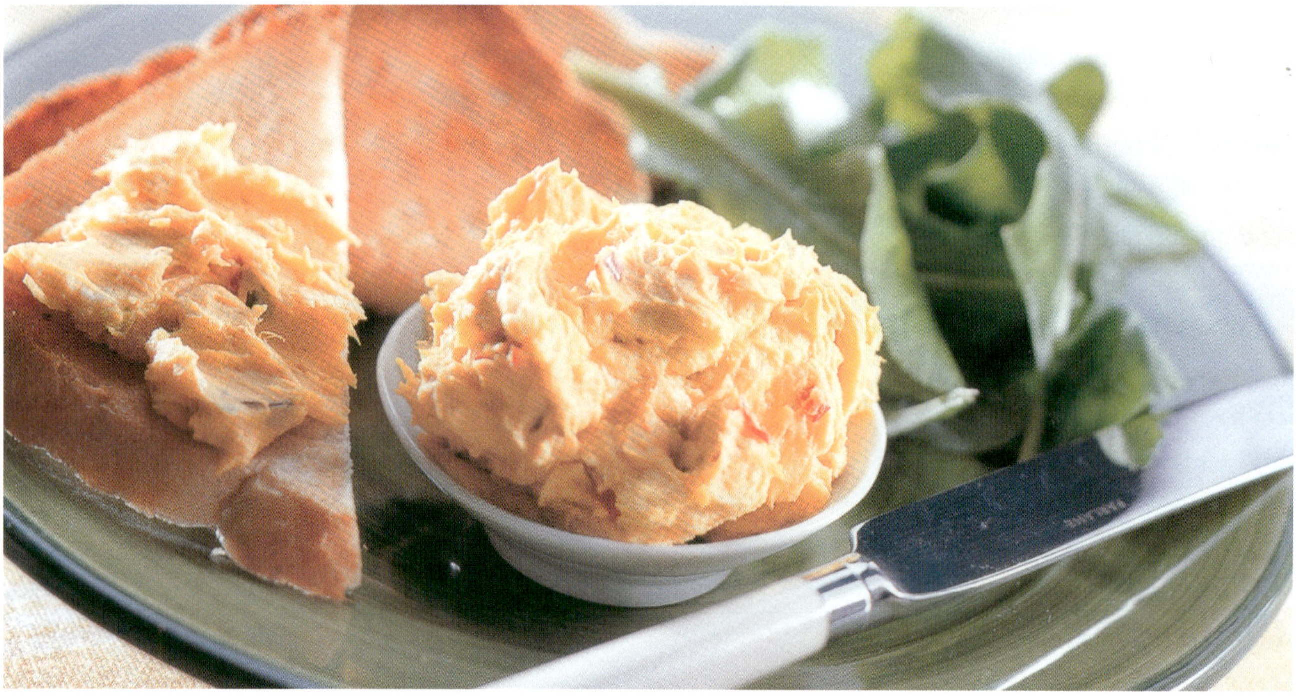

1 Preheat the oven to 220°C/gas mark 7. Cut the squash into 2.5 cm slices. Place them in a roasting pan, and season lightly. Drizzle with olive oil, then roast for 45 minutes. Leave the squash to cool, then cut the flesh away from the skin and mash it roughly.

NUTRITIONAL VALUES

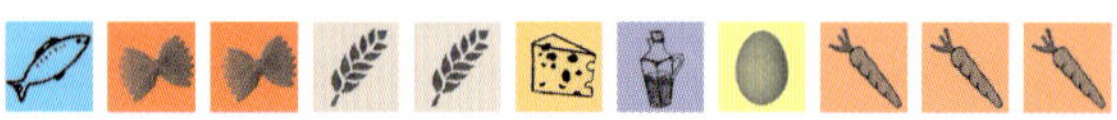

2 Beat the low-fat cream cheese with the garlic and chilli until smooth. Add the squash, mix together, then add the nuts, and season well. Turn into a serving dish and chill for 30 minutes.

3 Serve piled on hot slices of toast with a garnish of rocket leaves.

FRIED SARDINES

SERVES **4**

Sardines have a great flavour, and are beautifully complemented in this easy-to-prepare dish.

sardines (about 10 cm long)
75 g seasoned flour
freshly ground black pepper
olive oil to fry
lemon wedges, to serve

FOR THE MARINADE, BLEND TOGETHER

2 tsp parsley, chopped
4 tbsp lemon juice
1/2 tsp garlic, crushed
freshly ground black pepper
4 tbsp olive oil

INGREDIENTS FOR THE SAUCE/DIP

1 large tomato, skinned and chopped
2 small green peppers, deseeded and chopped
1/2 small onion, chopped
enough low-fat crème fraîche to bind
freshly ground black pepper

To prepare the sardines

1. Take the sardines (if the head is on, leave it) and cut through the bellies lengthways without cutting through the bone. Butterfly the fish.
2. Paint the marinade on the fish, and leave to marinate for 20 minutes.
3. Shake the flour over the fish, dusting until well covered. Shake off any excess flour. Season.
4. Heat the oil until hot and fry the sardines, turning to brown both sides.

To prepare the sauce/dip

1. Mix all the ingredients together, then either spoon onto plates with the sardines, or use as a dip.
2. Serve with lemon wedges.

NUTRITIONAL VALUES

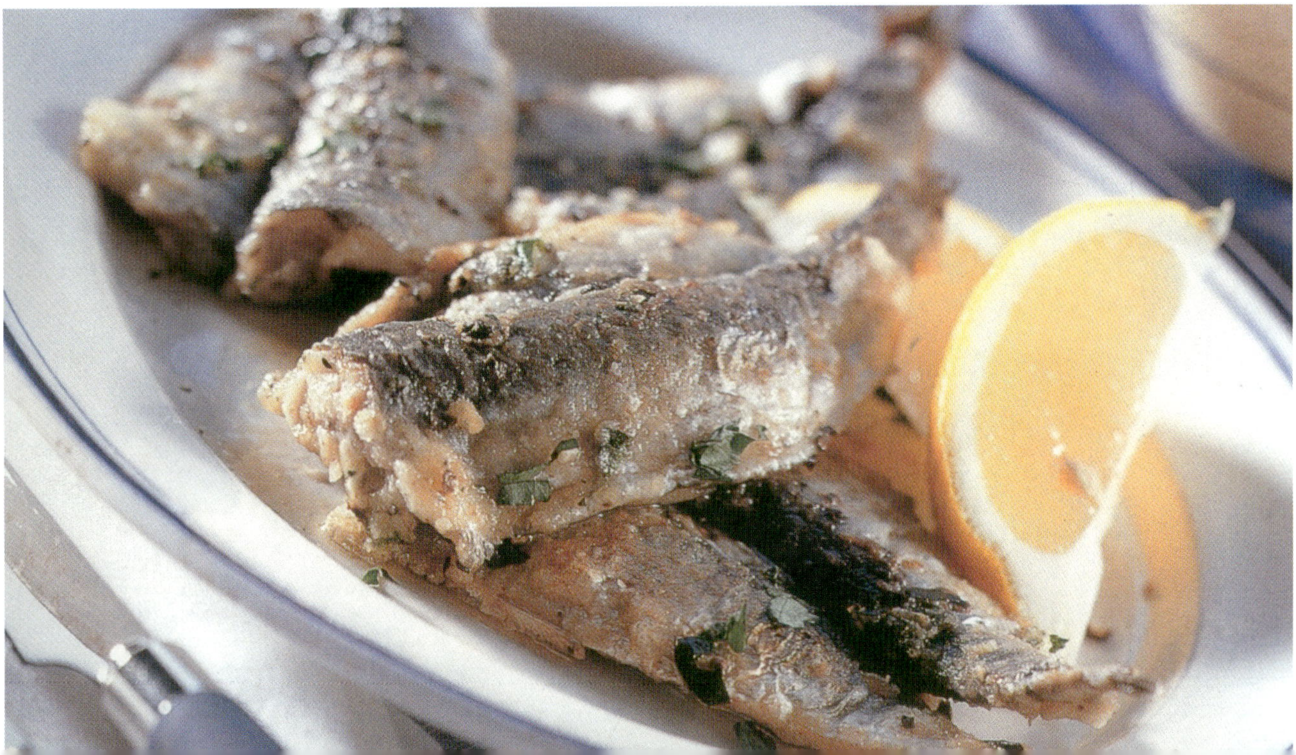

CRAB AND CORN PORRIDGE

SERVES **4**

If you want, fresh corn and crab can be used, but the recipe here saves time by using canned products. The result tastes just as good.

600 ml basic chicken stock or 1 can condensed cream of chicken soup
325 g can sweetcorn kernels
325 g can creamed corn
325 g can crabmeat, drained
1 egg
2 spring onions, cut into thin rings

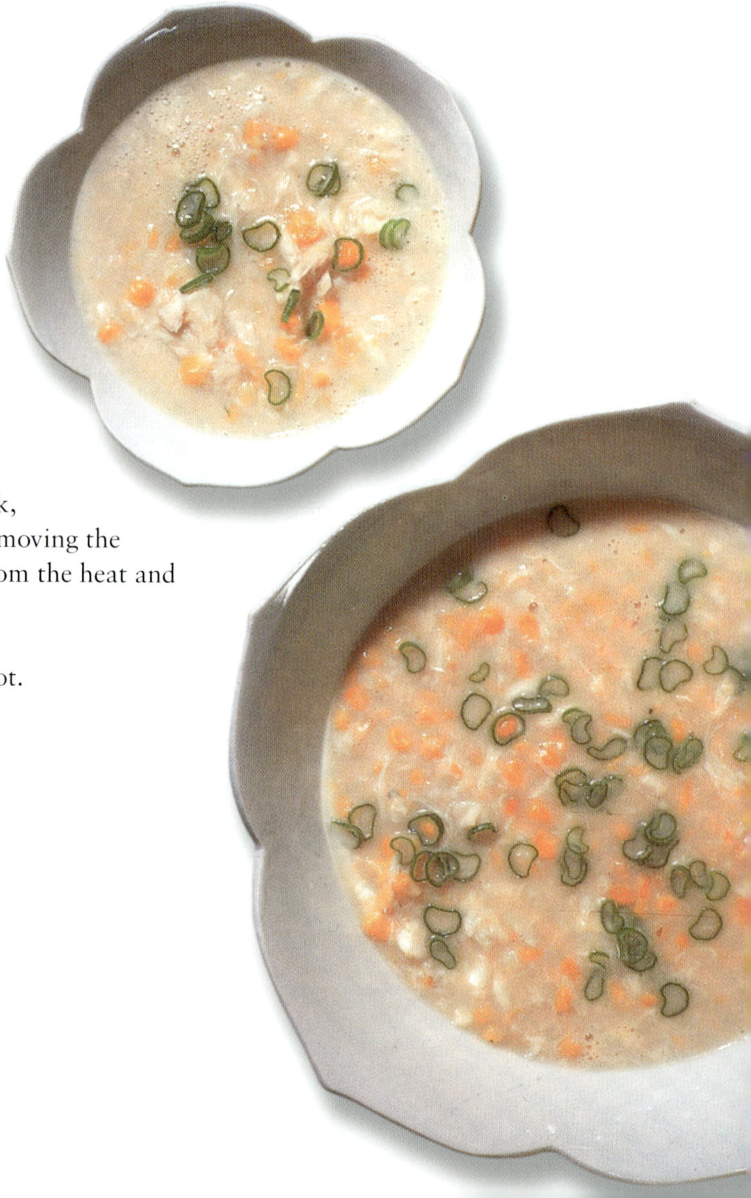

1 If using condensed soup, add 2 cans of water and milk mixed. Bring the stock or soup to just below boiling point.

2 Roughly chop the sweetcorn kernels or leave whole. Add the corn and the creamed corn to the stock. Add the crabmeat and stir thoroughly.

3 Beat the egg quickly and, holding a fork over the stock, pour the beaten egg along the back of the fork head, moving the fork in a circular motion at the same time. Remove from the heat and cover. Allow to set for about 40 seconds.

4 Sprinkle with the spring onions, stir once and serve hot.

NUTRITIONAL VALUES

BAKED STUFFED SWEET PEPPERS

SERVES **4**

When buying the sweet peppers, choose squat round peppers which still stand upright. Choose green, red, yellow or orange peppers, or even a mixture.

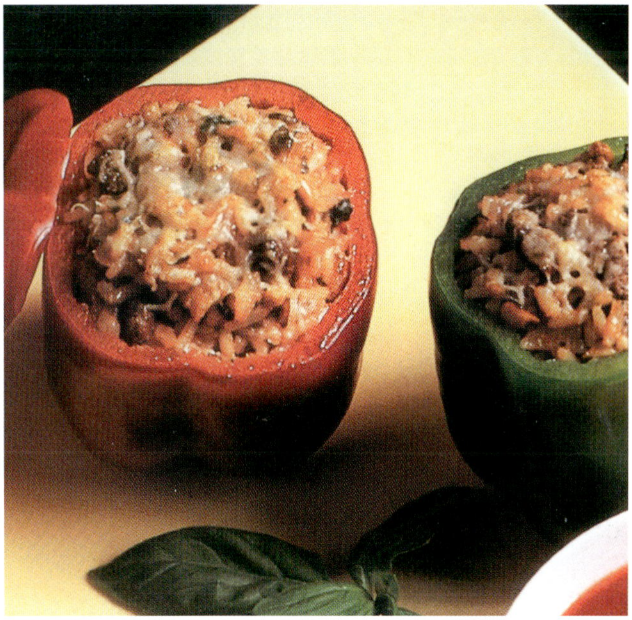

4 even-sized sweet peppers
2 tbsp olive oil
1 small onion, finely chopped
125 g long-grain rice
50 g button mushrooms, chopped
450 ml chicken stock (broth)
4 tbsp tomato purée
2 tbsp fresh basil, chopped
freshly ground black pepper
4–6 chicken livers, chopped
2 tbsp pinenuts, toasted
fresh basil leaves to garnish

1. Preheat the oven to oven to 180°C/gas mark 4. Cut the tops off the peppers and remove the cores and seeds. Put the peppers in a basin, cover with boiling water, and allow to stand for 5 minutes. Drain thoroughly and set aside.
2. Heat half the oil in a large pan and sauté the onion until softened. Stir in the rice and mushrooms and cook for a further minute; add the stock (broth), bring to the boil and simmer, covered, for 15 minutes, until the rice is just tender and the stock absorbed.
3. Stir in the tomato purée and the freshly chopped basil. Season to taste.
4. Heat the remaining oil and sauté the chicken livers until lightly browned. Stir into the rice with the pinenuts.
5. Spoon the rice mixture into the peppers and sprinkle them with the cheese.
6. Arrange the peppers in an ovenproof dish. Pour a little water into the dish (just enough to cover its base) and cook for 35 minutes or until the peppers are tender. Serve hot, garnished with fresh basil leaves.

NUTRITIONAL VALUES

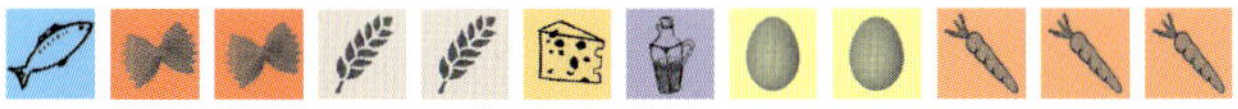

CHICKEN AND SPINACH TERRINE

SERVES **8–18**

A perfect start to a dinner party, or as a main course for a summer lunch. Serve on its own, or with new potatoes and a fresh crisp green salad.

SPINACH MIXTURE

500 g cooked spinach, well drained and chopped
freshly grated nutmeg
freshly ground black pepper
150 ml low-fat fromage frais
2 egg yolks
2 tsp powdered gelatine

CHICKEN MIXTURE

1 tbsp vegetable oil
700 g boneless chicken, minced
1 clove garlic, crushed
1 tsp green peppercorns
freshly ground black pepper
salt substitute (see page 18)
4 tbsp dry Vermouth
25 g pistachio nuts
175 ml low-fat fromage frais
3 tsp powdered gelatine

SAUCE

200 ml thick natural low-fat yogurt
1 bunch watercress, washed and trimmed
1 whole clove garlic, peeled
4 tbsp dry white wine
freshly ground black pepper

GARNISH

a few green peppercorns or a sprig of dill

1 For the spinach mixture, mix the spinach with nutmeg and pepper to taste. Blend in the low-fat fromage frais and egg yolks.

2 Dissolve the gelatine in 2 tablespoons water (place in a basin over a pan of simmering water). Allow to cool slightly before stirring into the spinach mixture.

3 For the chicken mixture, heat the oil and stir-fry the minced chicken for 4–5 minutes. Do not allow it to brown.

4 Add the garlic, green peppercorns, salt substitute and pepper to taste, and the Vermouth. Bubble briskly for 1 minute.

5 Blend the chicken in a liquidizer or food processor until smooth. Stir the pistachio nuts and fromage frais into the chicken mixture.

6 Dissolve the gelatine in 3 tablespoons water (as above) and add to the chicken mixture; blend well.

7 Put half the chicken mixture into a lightly oiled and lined 1 kg loaf tin, cover carefully with the spinach mixture, and spread the remaining chicken mixture over the top. Chill until the terrine is firm enough to slice.

8 Meanwhile, make the sauce. Put the yoghurt, watercress and garlic into a liquidizer or food processor and blend until smooth. Stir in the white wine and season to taste.

9 Carefully unmould the set terrine and cut into slices. Place a slice on each serving plate, and spoon a pool of sauce around the terrine. Garnish with a few extra green peppercorns or a sprig of fresh dill.

NUTRITIONAL VALUES

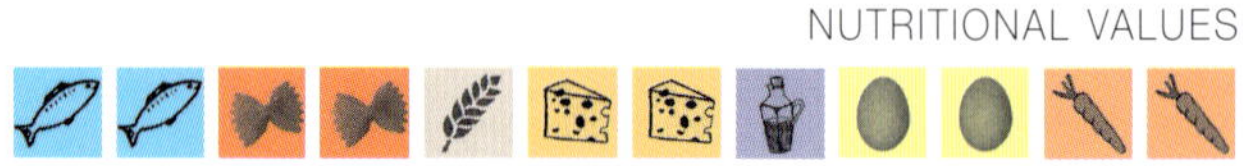

FUNGHI RIPIENI

SERVES **4**

This recipe for spinach-stuffed mushrooms is packed full of flavour and antioxidants, making it both a delicious and healthy starter.

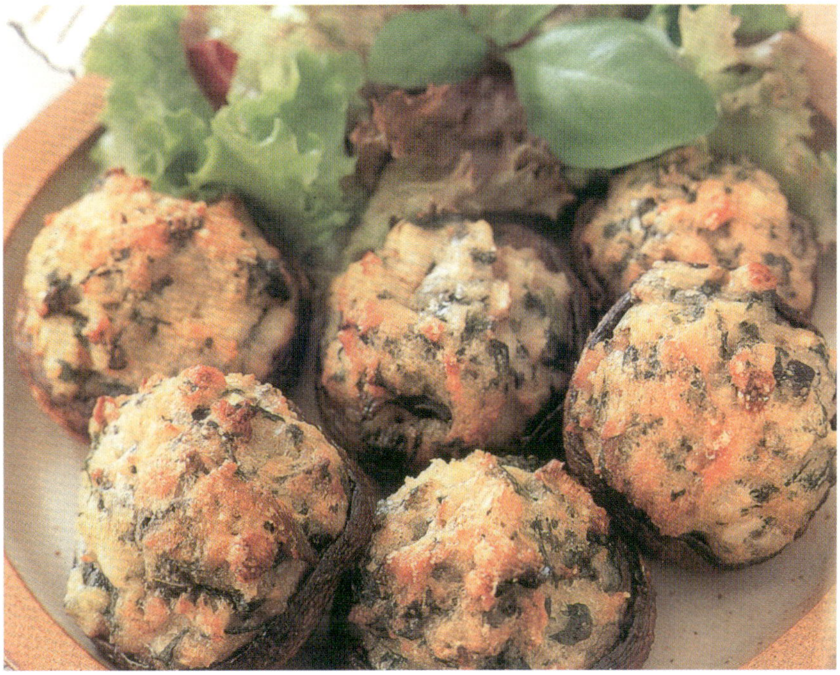

450 g firm, cultivated, open-cup mushrooms
40–65 g olive oil
3–5 garlic cloves, chopped
175 g cooked, chopped spinach
3–5 spring onions, thinly sliced
2–3 tsp fresh marjoram, basil, thyme and/or rosemary
75 g freshly grated Parmesan or pecorino cheese, plus a little extra for sprinkling
1 egg, lightly beaten
wholemeal breadcrumbs, for binding
freshly ground black pepper

1 Preheat the oven to 190°C/gas mark 5 oven. Break the stalks off all the mushrooms and chop finely. In the oil, lightly sauté the mushroom stalks with the garlic, then add the spinach, spring onions and fresh herbs. Remove from the heat and mix in the remaining ingredients, using just enough breadcrumbs to hold the mixture together. If the filling doesn't seem mushroomy enough, take a few of the mushroom caps, chop finely, and add to the filling.

2 Arrange the caps on a baking sheet and fill each one with the filling, pressing it in firmly. Sprinkle with cheese, then bake for 10–15 minutes, or until the mushrooms are juicy and the cheese lightly browned. Serve immediately.

NUTRITIONAL VALUES

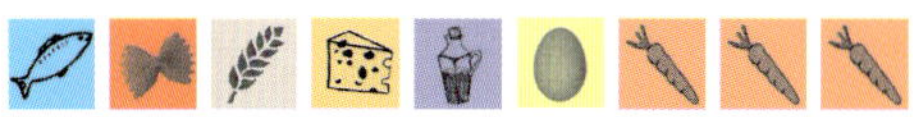

SUN-DRIED TOMATOES & YELLOW PEPPERS

SERVES **4**

This starter is delicious on small pieces of French bread or crisp crostini-like toasts.

3 yellow peppers, cut into bite-sized pieces
4–5 tbsp extra virgin olive oil
4–5 garlic cloves, finely chopped
400 g ripe tomatoes, diced
freshly ground black pepper
8–10 marinated sun-dried tomatoes, cut into quarters
1 tbsp balsamic vinegar or to taste
2–3 capers, rinsed and drained
chopped parsley, to garnish

NUTRITIONAL VALUES

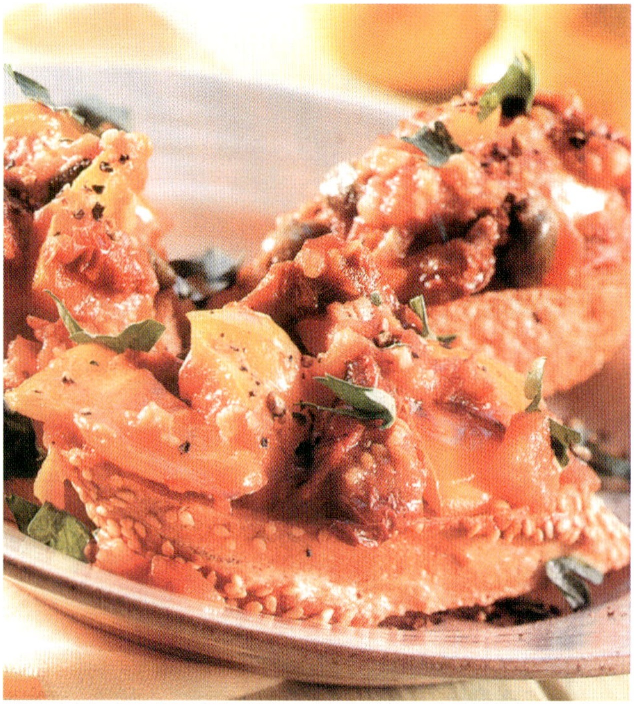

1 Sauté the peppers in the olive oil for about 7 minutes until lightly brown but not too soft. Add half the garlic, the tomatoes, and seasoning, and cook over high heat until the tomatoes reduce to a thick paste.

2 Stir in the sun-dried tomatoes, balsamic vinegar, capers and remaining garlic. Let cool to room temperature to serve. Garnish with parsley.

MAIN COURSES

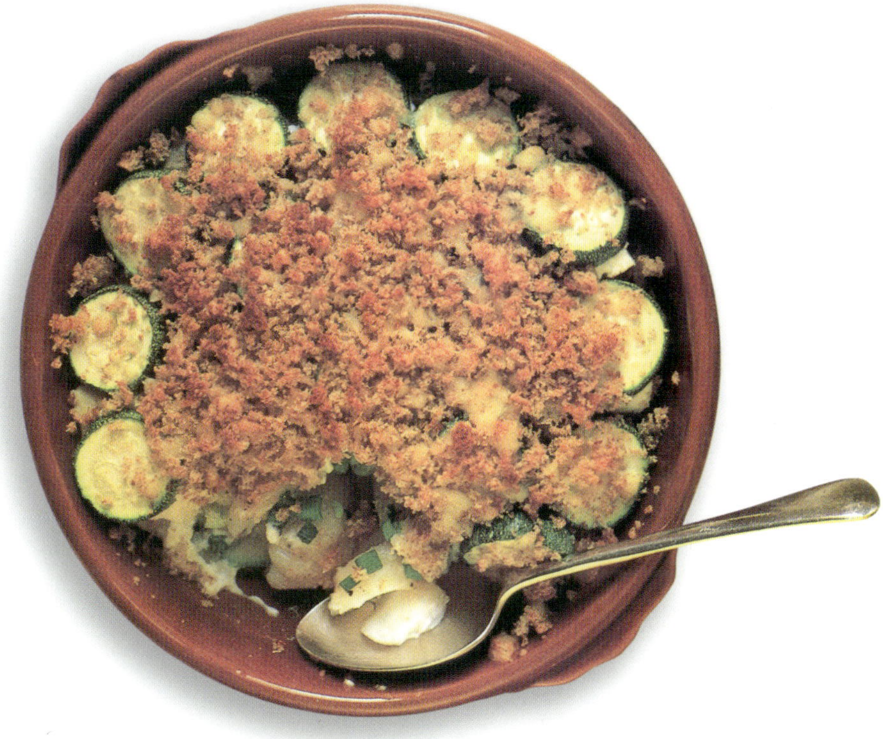

ROBIN'S VEGETARIAN CHILLI WITH PEACHES AND THREE BEANS

SERVES **12**

This is a meatless chilli, which originates from Orlando, Florida. Instead of using a meat substitute, peaches are used to make a sweet and delicious meal.

1 red pepper, coarsely chopped
2 green peppers, coarsely chopped
1 large onion, coarsely chopped
1 peach, peeled and coarsely chopped
2 x 400 g cans tomatoes, coarsely chopped
2 x 400 g cans tomato sauce
1 tsp Tabasco sauce
1/4 tsp dried thyme
1 tsp dried oregano
2 tsp ground cumin, or more to taste
1 tbsp chilli powder
1 tsp black pepper
2 x 300 g cans cannelloni beans
2 x 450 g cans black beans
450 g can kidney beans

1 Put all the ingredients, except the beans, in a stockpot with about 250 ml water and stir well. Bring to the boil, reduce heat and simmer for 30 minutes, stirring often to avoid scorching, and adding water if needed.

2 After 30 minutes, add the beans and enough liquid for the desired consistency. Simmer for 15 minutes more. Taste and adjust seasonings.

NUTRITIONAL VALUES

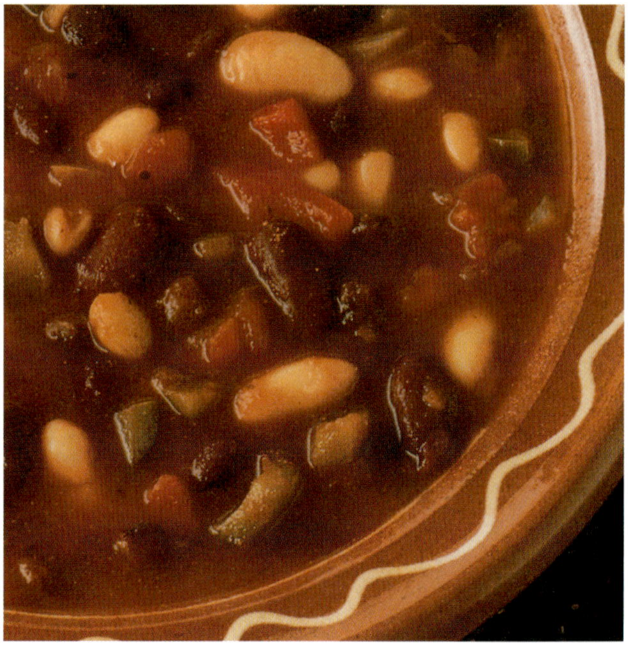

INTERALLIA

SERVES **4–6**

This dish is so named because it combines five of the allium family in one delicious vegetable mixture.

- 3 heads unpeeled garlic (about 35 cloves)
- 350 g baby onions
- 4 tbsp olive oil
- 350 g young leeks, trimmed and cut into 2.5 cm chunks
- 100 ml water
- 25 g flour
- $\frac{1}{2}$ tsp English mustard
- $\frac{1}{4}$ tsp turmeric
- 150 ml hot milk
- 3 tbsp low-fat crème fraîche
- freshly ground black pepper

TO SERVE

- 1 tbsp finely chopped spring onions (green part only)
- 1 tbsp chives, finely chopped

1. Separate the garlic cloves and blanch them together with the onions in boiling water for a couple of minutes. Drain and peel. Cook them very gently in half the oil for 7–10 minutes, then add the leeks and the water. Bring to the boil and set to one side.
2. Warm the remaining oil in a small saucepan, add the flour, mustard and turmeric, and stir for a few minutes. Turn up the heat, strain the liquid from the vegetables into it and add the hot milk. Simmer for 5 minutes. Pour over the vegetables and continue to simmer until they are just tender.
3. Remove from the heat and gently stir in the crème fraîche, and season with pepper to taste.
4. Sprinkle with the spring onions and the chives. This dish is especially good with grilled lean chicken and lamb.

NUTRITIONAL VALUES

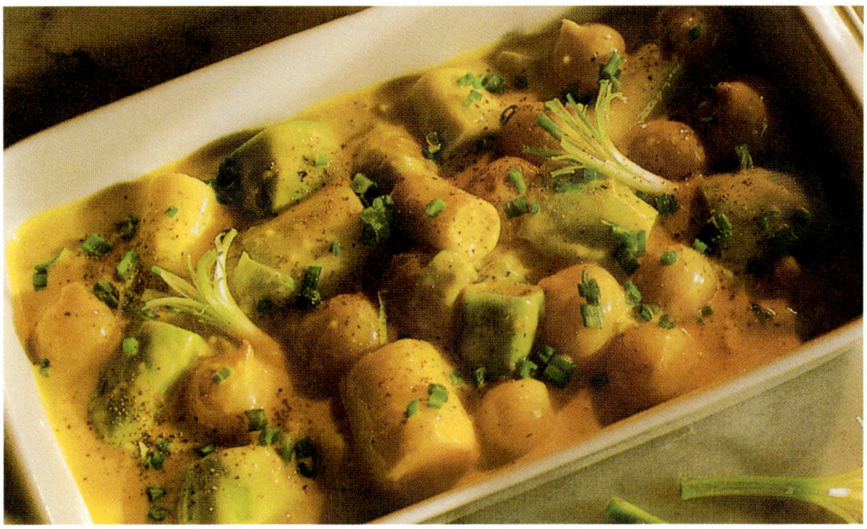

WARM BEAN AND PUMPKIN SALAD

SERVES **6**

Ideal for making in a slow cooker, the spinach cooks so quickly that it is added right at the very end of the cooking time. You could use frozen spinach, but fresh is definitely better. For a change, use Swiss chard in place of the spinach.

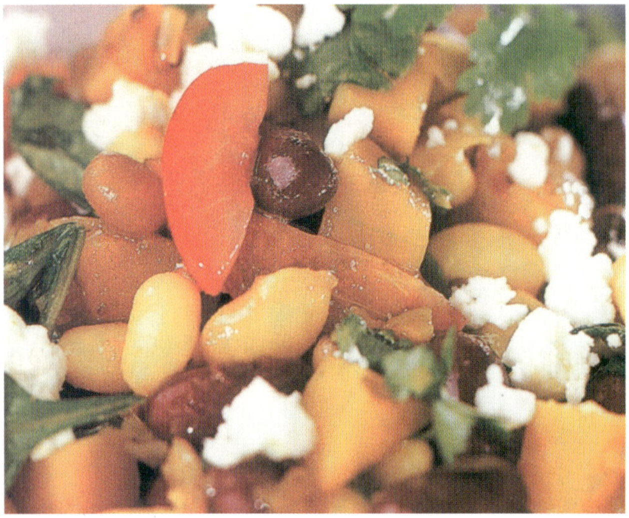

100 g dried haricot beans, soaked overnight
100 g dried red kidney beans, soaked overnight
100 g dried black-eye beans, soaked overnight
2 tbsp olive oil
1 large onion, peeled and cut into wedges
small piece fresh root ginger, peeled and shredded
2–4 garlic cloves, peeled and chopped
1/4–1 tsp dried crushed chilies
1 tsp cumin seeds
1 tsp ground coriander
1/2 tsp turmeric
450 g pumpkin, peeled, deseeded and diced
300 ml vegetable stock
100 g cherry tomatoes, quartered
175 g spinach, thoroughly washed and shredded
175 g feta cheese, diced
fresh coriander sprigs
freshly ground black pepper
low-fat natural yoghurt and warm pitta bread strips to serve

1 Cover the beans with cold water and leave to soak overnight. Next day, drain, place in a pan and cover with water. Bring to the boil and boil for 10 minutes. Drain and reserve.

2 Preheat the slow cooker on high. Heat the oil in a frying pan and sauté the onion with the ginger, garlic, chillies to taste and all the spices for 3 minutes. Add the pumpkin and continue to sauté for 3 more minutes, then spoon into the cooking pot and stir in the drained beans. Heat the stock to boiling and pour over the vegetables and beans. Cover, reduce temperature to low, then cook for 8–10 hours.

3 Just before serving, stir in the tomatoes and spinach, stir well and continue to cook for 15–20 minutes or until the spinach has begun to wilt. Sprinkle with the diced feta cheese and the freshly chopped coriander and serve with low-fat yoghurt and strips of warm pitta bread.

NUTRITIONAL VALUES

CELLOPHANE NOODLES WITH VEGETABLES

SERVES **4**

This is a colourful, vegetable-packed noodle dish with a multitude of different textures. Once the vegetables have been prepared it is remarkably quick to assemble and cook.

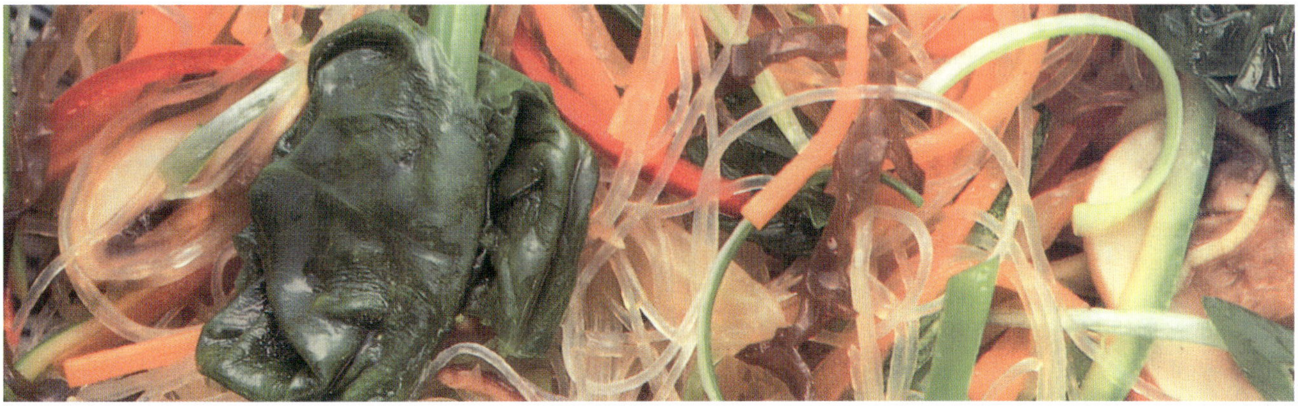

- 6 dried Chinese black mushrooms, soaked in hot water for 30 minutes
- 150 g young fresh spinach leaves
- 2 Chinese cabbage leaves
- 3 shiitake or oyster mushrooms, thinly sliced
- 4 spring onions, white or green parts thickly sliced diagonally
- 1 small courgette, cut into fine strips
- 1 carrot, cut into fine strips
- 4 tbsp olive oil
- 1 tbsp sesame oil
- 3 garlic cloves, crushed and finely chopped
- 2 small fresh red chillies, deseeded and cut into fine strips
- 50 g cellophane noodles or vermicelli noodles, soaked for 30 minutes and drained
- 1 tbsp soy sauce

NUTRITIONAL VALUES

1 Drain the dried mushrooms and cut away and discard the stems and any hard parts. Thinly slice the mushroom caps.

2 Add the spinach to a large saucepan of boiling water. Cover and quickly return to the boil. Boil for 2 minutes then drain and rinse under running cold water. Drain well and squeeze out as much water as possible. Separate the leaves.

3 Cut away and discard the curly outer part of the Chinese cabbage leaves, saving only the 'V' shaped core of the leaves. Cut this into fine strips then mix with the spinach, dried and fresh mushrooms, spring onions, courgette and carrot until well mixed.

4 Heat the olive oil and sesame oil in a deep frying pan, add the garlic and chilli and stir-fry for 10 seconds. Add the mixed vegetables and stir-fry for 3–4 minutes until the vegetables are tender but still crisp. Turn the heat to low and stir in the noodles and soy sauce. Cook for 2 minutes then serve.

PASTA-STUFFED CABBAGE LEAVES

SERVES **4**

Easy to prepare and sure to impress the guests, this dish can be made the day before and kept in the refrigerator. Allow an extra 15–20 minutes to reheat in the oven before serving.

NUTRITIONAL VALUES

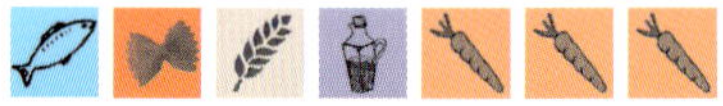

75 g dried pastina (any tiny shapes)

dash of olive oil

8 large savoy cabbage leaves, stalks removed

FOR THE FILLING

2 tbsp olive oil

2 cloves garlic, crushed

2 carrots, grated

2 courgettes, grated

4 tomatoes, skinned, deseeded and chopped

55 g chopped walnuts

freshly ground black pepper

FOR THE SAUCE

400 g can chopped tomatoes

4 tbsp dry red wine

150 ml vegetable stock

1 tbsp dried oregano

1 onion, very finely chopped

freshly ground black pepper

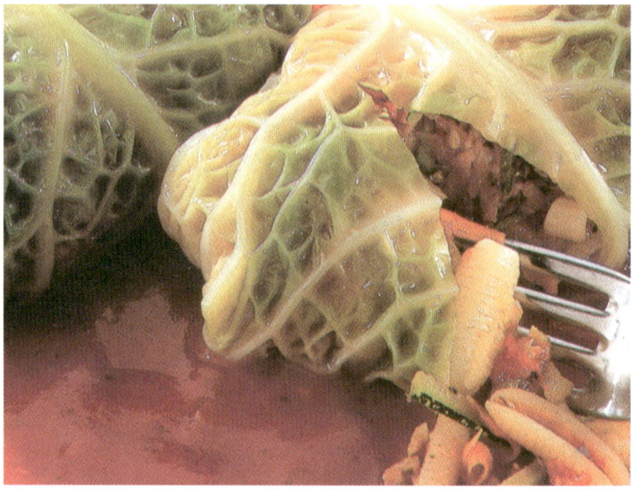

1 Bring a large saucepan of water to the boil and add the pasta with a dash of olive oil. Cook for about 10 minutes, stirring occasionally, until tender. Drain and set aside.

2 Blanch the cabbage leaves in boiling water, then quickly immerse in cold water and drain. Pat dry with absorbent kitchen paper and set aside.

3 To make the filling, heat the olive oil in a large frying pan and sauté the garlic for about 1 minute. Add the grated carrots and courgettes and cook for a further 3–4 minutes, stirring occasionally, until tender.

4 Add the chopped tomatoes, walnuts and pasta. Season with freshly ground black pepper. Cook for about 5 minutes, stirring occasionally, then set aside to cool.

5 To make the sauce, place all the ingredients in a saucepan and bring to simmering point. Cook for 20–30 minutes, stirring occasionally, until reduced and thickened. Allow to cool slightly, then transfer to a food processor or blender and purée until smooth. Set aside. Preheat the oven to 200°C/gas mark 6.

6 To assemble the stuffed cabbage leaves, lay the blanched leaves out on the work surface, concave side uppermost, and divide the mixture among the leaves, placing it in the centre of each. Fold the edge of each leaf over to completely encase the filling, securing it with a cocktail stick.

7 Arrange the stuffed leaves in a shallow ovenproof dish and pour the sauce around the edges. Cover with aluminium foil and bake for about 20 minutes, until heated through. Serve immediately, with any extra sauce served separately.

MACKEREL WITH SPICY TOMATO JAM

SERVES **4**

Mackerel is a very oily, medium-firm fish that contains a high level of vitamin A, so this comforting dish is very good for you. The tomatoes add bite to the dish, as well as high levels of antioxidants.

450 g tomatoes, skinned, deseeded and chopped
1 medium Spanish onion, diced
125 ml apple jelly
50 ml cider vinegar
1 tbsp chopped tarragon
1 tsp salt substitute (see page 18)
$\frac{1}{2}$–1 tsp crushed red chilli pepper
4 x 225 g mackerel fillets, cleaned, with heads removed but with skin left on
olive oil
freshly ground black pepper, to taste
tarragon sprigs and orange slices, to garnish

1 Combine the tomato, onion, jelly, vinegar, tarragon, and red chilli pepper in a medium saucepan. Bring to the boil over a medium-high heat. Reduce the heat to medium-low and cook, stirring frequently, 35–45 minutes or until thick. Cool the jam to room temperature.

2 Season the mackerel with pepper and brush the skin with olive oil. Grill, skin side down, covered, over medium-hot heat, 5 minutes on each side. Do not turn the fish or overcook it.

3 To serve, top each fillet with 2 tablespoons of tomato jam and season to taste. Garnish with tarragon and orange slices.

NUTRITIONAL VALUES

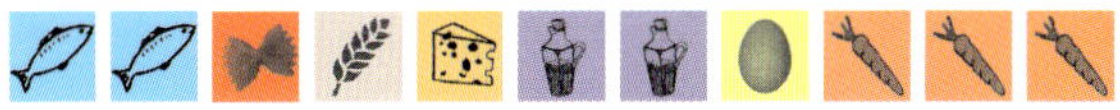

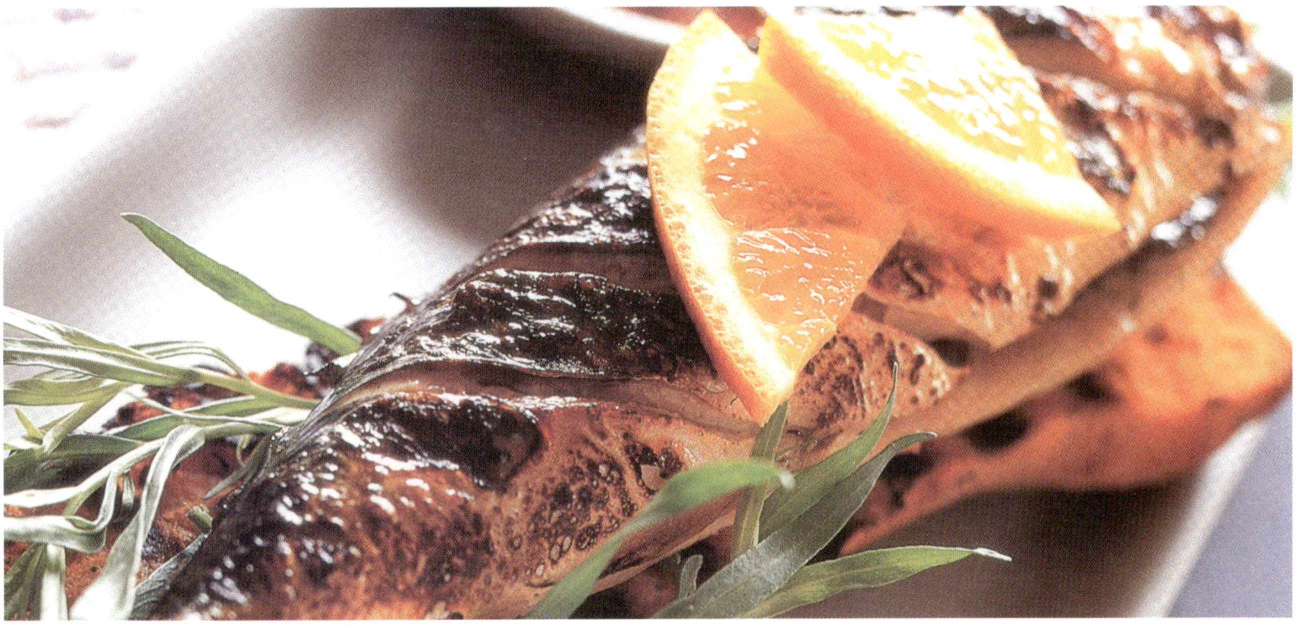

GRILLED TUNA WITH ORANGE, THYME AND GARLIC

SERVES **6**

The flavours of orange and tuna complement each other wonderfully well. In this recipe, thin slices of garlic are pushed into the tuna steaks, creating an intensely garlicky dish.

juice of 1 large orange
3 plump garlic cloves, very thinly sliced
2 tbsp fresh thyme leaves
1 tbsp finely grated orange rind
salt substitute (see page 18) and freshly ground black pepper
6 tuna steaks, about 2.5 cm thick

NUTRITIONAL VALUES

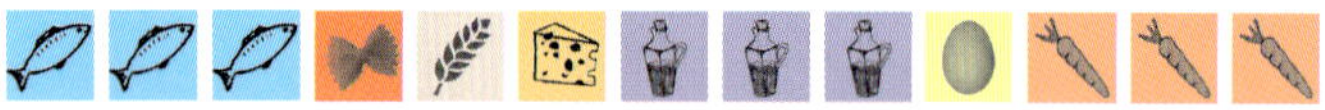

1 Put the orange juice, garlic, thyme, orange rind and seasoning into a shallow non-metallic dish, large enough to hold the tuna in a single layer. Mix well, then add the tuna steaks, turning them until evenly coated. Push some of the garlic slices between the flakes of the tuna.

2 Cover and leave to marinate in the refrigerator for 30 minutes–1 hour, turning the tuna once or twice during this time.

3 Lift the fish out of its marinade and cook over medium-high heat for about 4–5 minutes on each side or until very nearly cooked through.

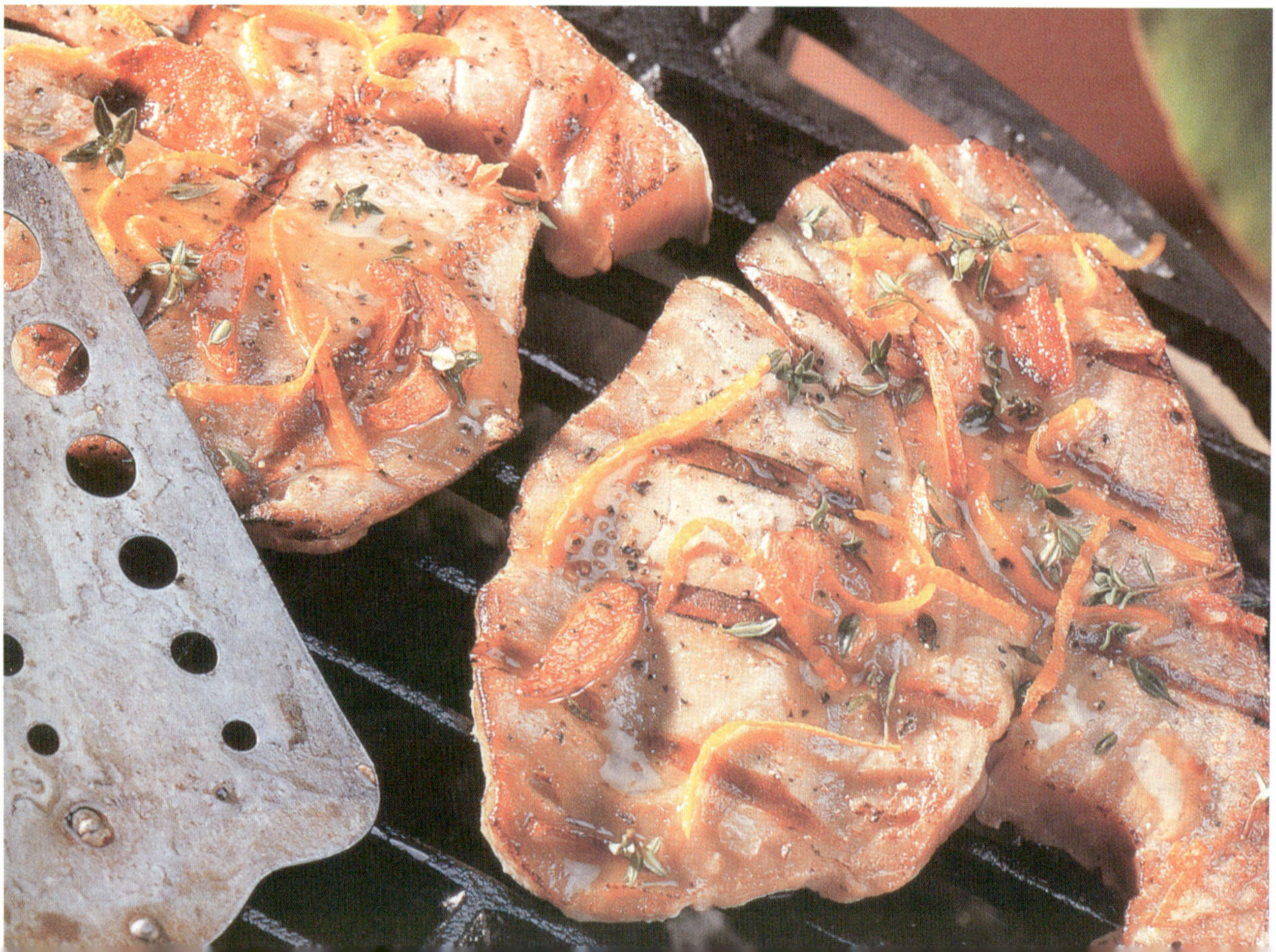

FISH AND VEGETABLE CASSEROLE

SERVES **8–10**

Cod, haddock and monkfish are each suitable types of fish to use for this dish, which originates from the Greek island of Corfu. The crucial ingredient is the garlic, and plenty of it.

7 tbsp olive oil
1 large onion, sliced
900 g small new potatoes, washed and cut into 1.2 cm slices
2 carrots, cut into 2.5 cm chunks
1 celery stick, chopped
salt substitute (see page 18) and freshly ground black pepper
6 garlic cloves, crushed
1.12 kg firm white fish fillets, skinned and cut into 5 cm chunks
63 ml freshly squeezed lemon juice

NUTRITIONAL VALUES

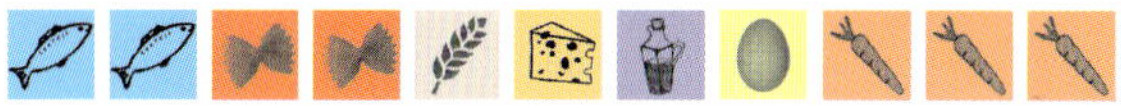

1 Heat 4 tablespoons of the olive oil in a large, heavy-based saucepan and sauté the onion for about 3 minutes, or until softened.

2 Add the potatoes, carrots and celery, and season with salt substitute and freshly ground black pepper. Continue to cook for a further 4–5 minutes, or until the vegetables begin to soften.

3 Stir in the garlic and pour over enough boiling water to just cover the vegetables. Bring to the boil, cover and simmer for 10–15 minutes or until the vegetables are almost tender.

4 Gently stir the fish into the casserole, cover and simmer for 10–15 minutes or until the fish flakes easily, adding a little extra water if necessary. Just before the end of the cooking time, remove the cover and stir in the lemon juice and the remaining olive oil. Adjust the seasoning if necessary and serve.

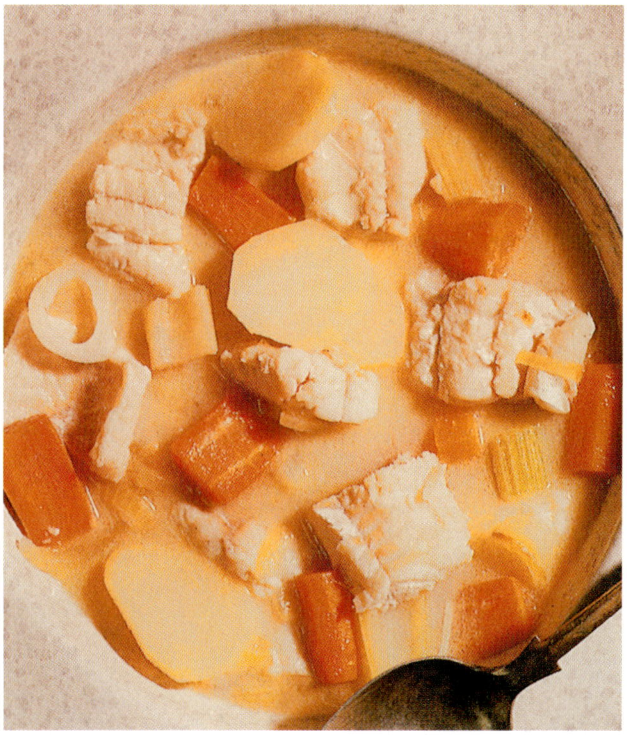

COD AND COURGETTE GRATIN

SERVES **4**

You can substitute any white fish for the cod – try strips of flounder fillet, or chunks of haddock. Smoked fish – haddock, cod or coley fillet – are also particularly flavoursome.

450 g courgettes, trimmed and sliced
675 g cod fillet, skinned, and cut into chunks
2 tbsp chopped fresh parsley
2 tbsp chopped fresh tarragon, or 1 tbsp dried tarragon
4 tbsp snipped chives or chopped spring onions
salt substitute (see page 18) and freshly ground black pepper
125 g low-fat cream cheese
60 g fresh wholemeal breadcrumbs
125 g grated Cheddar cheese

NUTRITIONAL VALUES

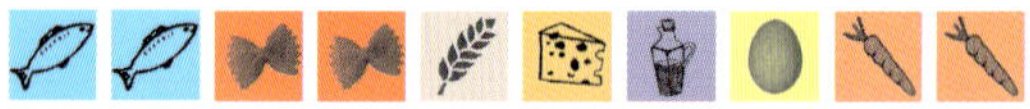

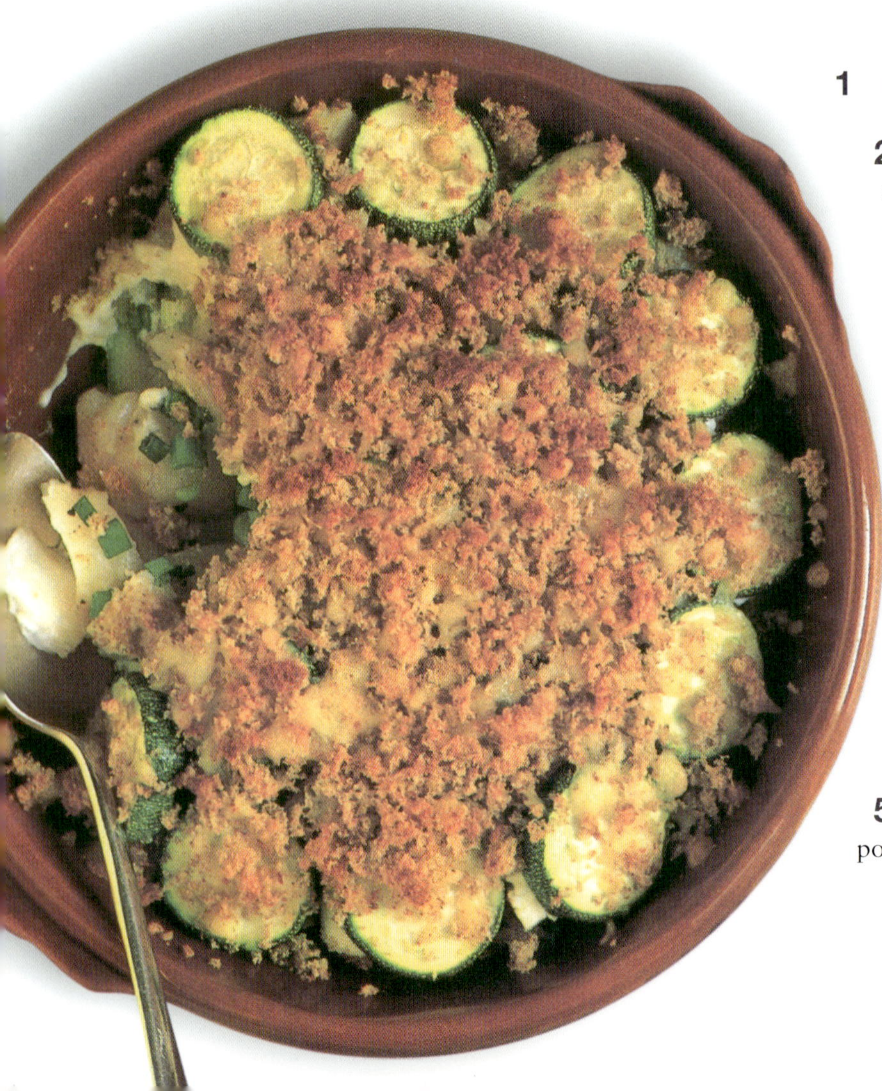

1 Preheat the oven to 180°C/gas mark 4.

2 Arrange half the courgettes in the base of a shallow dish – a gratin dish is ideal, a quiche dish is too shallow, and a casserole will do.

3 Make sure there are no bones in the fish, then place it on top of the courgettes. Sprinkle the parsley, tarragon and chives or spring onions over. Season well, then dot with the cream cheese. Top with the remaining courgettes.

4 Mix the breadcrumbs with the Cheddar cheese, then sprinkle the mixture over the courgette. Bake for about 1 hour, until the topping is golden and the courgettes are just tender. Under the topping, the fish and lower layer of courgettes are baked in a herby, creamy sauce.

5 Serve at once, with baked or mashed potatoes, or a bowl of freshly cooked pasta.

ONION RAVIOLI WITH WALNUT AND SORREL SAUCE

SERVES **2**

This is a rich and delicious pasta dish. Serve it as a main course with a simple side salad, or divide into smaller portions and serve as an appetizer.

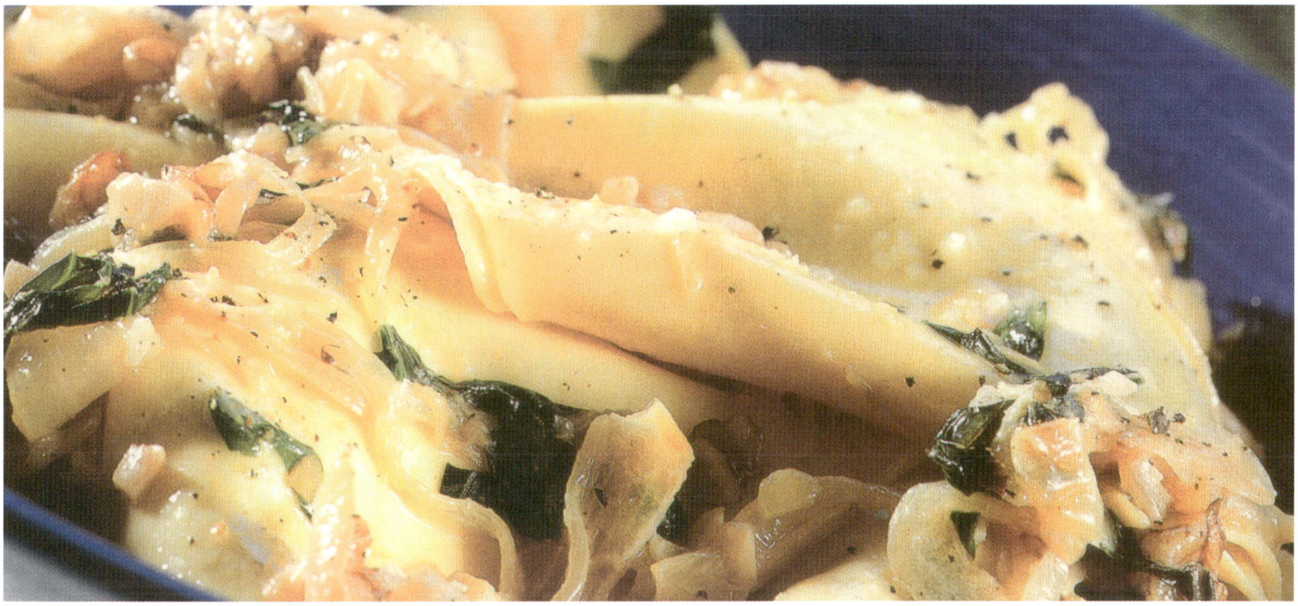

2 large onions
4 tbsp olive oil
1 clove garlic, finely chopped
large pinch ground mace
freshly ground black pepper
12 fresh no-cook lasagne noodles
62 g chopped walnuts
8 tbsp olive oil
1–2 tbsp shredded sorrel

NUTRITIONAL VALUES

1. Chop $1^{1}/_{2}$ of the onions, then cook them in the olive oil with the garlic and mace until soft and golden brown – about 10 minutes over a medium heat. Add pepper and allow to cool.

2. Dampen the edges and crossways along the middle of each sheet of lasagne, one at a time. Place about 1 teaspoon of onions on one end of each noodle, then fold the lasagne over in half and seal the edges to make a ravioli pouch. Leave on a damp tea towel until ready to cook.

3. Slice the remaining onion and cook it in the pan until golden with any remaining onion filling. Once browned, add the chopped walnuts and the oil. Heat until the nuts have browned and then keep warm.

4. Bring a large pan of water to a boil. Add the ravioli and cook gently for 3–4 minutes, then drain and add to the sauce with the shredded sorrel. Season to taste and serve.

CORIANDER CHICKEN WITH PILAU RICE

SERVES **4**

Fresh coriander has a unique, pungent flavour and goes perfectly with chicken.

1 tbsp olive oil
8 chicken thighs
1 large onion, sliced
1 tsp paprika
1 tsp ground cumin
1 tsp turmeric
$\frac{1}{2}$ tsp dried thyme
freshly ground black pepper
300 ml well-flavoured chicken stock
25 g pitted black olives
2 tbsp fresh coriander, finely chopped
squeeze lemon juice

PILAU RICE

2 tbsp olive oil
50 g whole blanched almonds, toasted
1 small onion, finely diced
50 g sultanas or raisins
375 g long-grain rice
750 ml boiling water

1. Heat the oil in a large pan and fry the chicken until an even, rich brown. Transfer to a plate.
2. Add the onion to the remaining oil and cook until softened and golden. Stir in the paprika, cumin and turmeric and cook for a further minute. Add the thyme, black pepper and stock and bring to the boil.
3. Return the chicken to the pan, skin side down. Cover and simmer for 1–$1\frac{1}{4}$ hours or until the chicken is tender.
4. Remove the chicken with a slotted spoon to a heated serving dish and keep warm.
5. Reduce the sauce by rapidly boiling until it thickens. Stir in the olives, coriander and lemon juice. Season to taste and pour over the chicken.
6. For the rice, heat the oil in a large pan and cook the onion until softened but not coloured. Add the toasted almonds, sultanas and rice, and cook for a further minute, stirring thoroughly.
7. Add the boiling water and bring to the boil, then cover and reduce the heat to a simmer. Cook for 15 minutes, or until all the water has been absorbed and the rice is tender, but still firm. Fork the rice lightly and serve with the chicken.

NUTRITIONAL VALUES

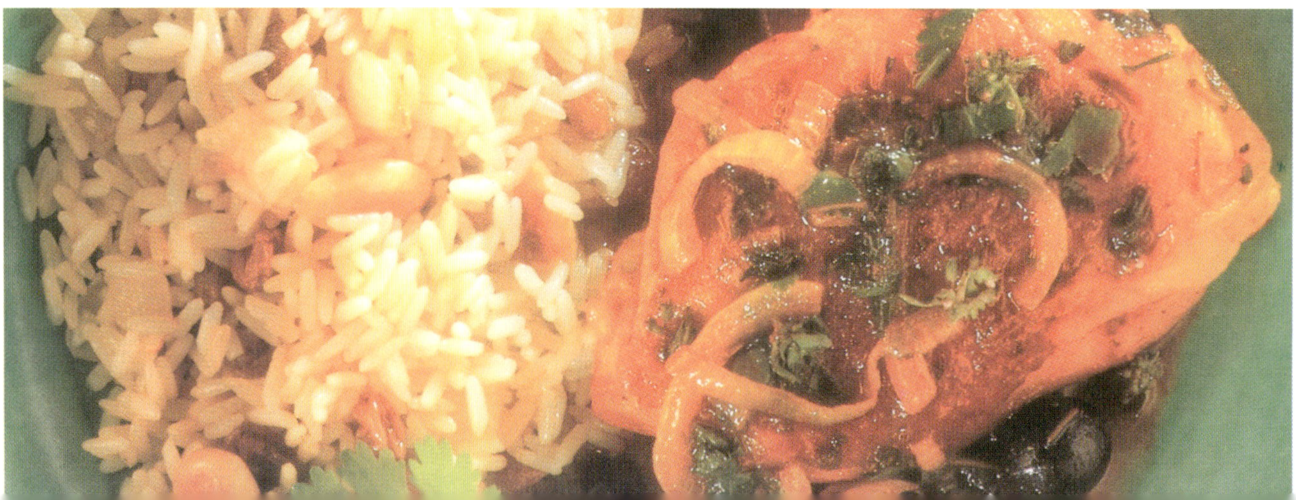

TROUT WITH WILD RICE STUFFING

SERVES **4**

Wild rice makes excellent stuffings. It goes well with game birds such as pheasant and duck, or with fish. Do not mix the stuffing with egg when using it with fish, as a crumbly stuffing seems to go better with the flaky fish texture.

4 trout, brown or rainbow

STUFFING

1 small onion, finely chopped

1 stick celery, finely sliced

1 tbsp olive oil

$^1/_2$ small green pepper, finely chopped

1 clove garlic, crushed

150 g cooked wild rice (about 50 g raw)

1 tbsp freshly chopped dill or parsley

1 lemon, grated rind and juice

freshly ground black pepper

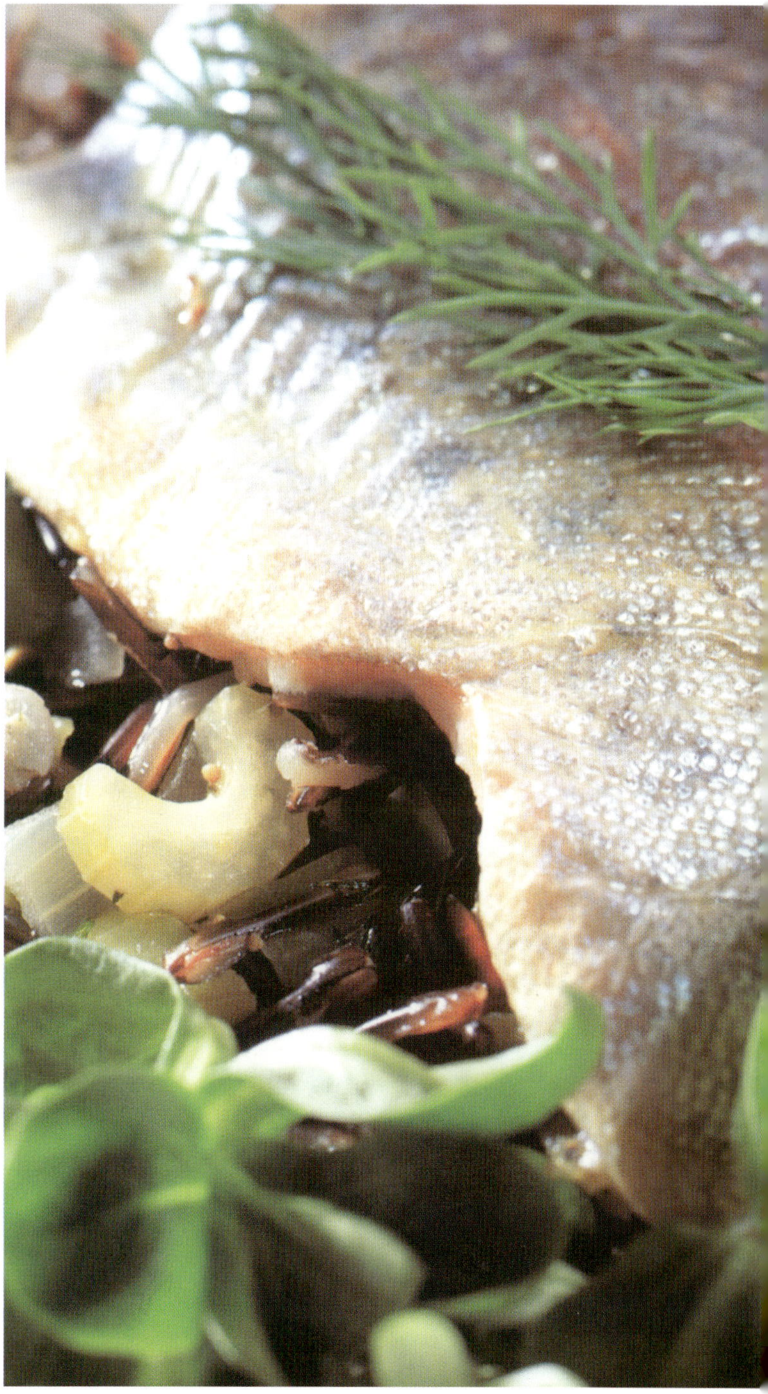

NUTRITIONAL VALUES

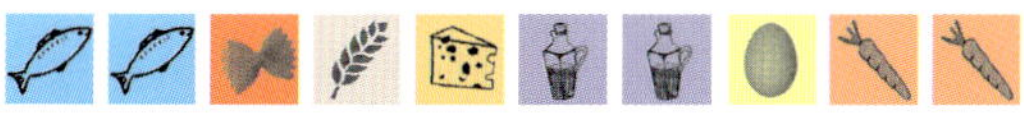

1 Preheat the oven to 200°C/gas mark 6. Lightly oil a suitable ovenproof dish.

2 Cook the onion and celery in the olive oil until softened but not browned. Add the pepper and continue cooking until all the vegetables are soft. Remove the pan from the heat and stir in the garlic and cooked rice. Add the herbs, lemon rind and juice, then season to taste with freshly ground black pepper.

3 Clean the trout, removing the heads if preferred. Season the cavities of the fish with the peppper and fill with the stuffing. Arrange the fish in the prepared dish and cover with foil. Bake for 15–20 minutes, according to the size of the fish, until just cooked. Serve immediately while still hot.

POACHED SALMON FILLETS WITH DILL AND GINGER VINAIGRETTE

SERVES **4**

Salmon has great colour and flavour that goes extremely well with this dill and ginger vinaigrette.

4 boneless salmon fillets, 175 g each, with skin on
9 large sprigs fresh dill
1 bay leaf
4 whole cloves
9 whole black peppercorns
2 tbsp white wine vinegar

DILL AND GINGER VINAIGRETTE
2 tbsp French mustard
1 tbsp grated root ginger
2 tbsp finely chopped shallot
1 tsp finely chopped garlic
2 tbsp tarragon vinegar
50 g canned pimentos, diced
freshly ground black pepper
125 ml olive oil

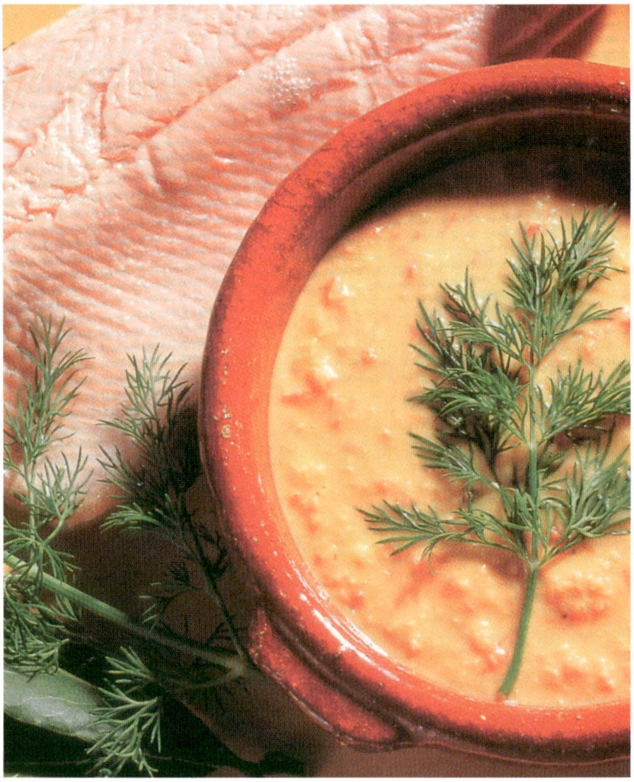

1 Prepare the vinaigrette by whisking the mustard, ginger, shallot, garlic, vinegar, pimentos and pepper together in a bowl. Then add the olive oil in a slow stream, whisking rapidly until well blended. Set aside.

2 Place the salmon fillets in a shallow saucepan with enough water to cover. Add all but one dill sprig, the bay leaf, cloves, peppercorns and vinegar. Bring the water to the boil and simmer for 3–5 minutes. Do not overcook. Drain and serve with the vinaigrette, giving the vinaigrette a last-second whisking, if necessary. Float the reserved sprig of dill on top of the bowl of vinaigrette.

NUTRITIONAL VALUES

GRILLED SARDINES WITH SPAGHETTI SQUASH

SERVES **4**

This is an easy-to-prepare dish that is full of flavour and is high in antioxidants, protein and fibre.

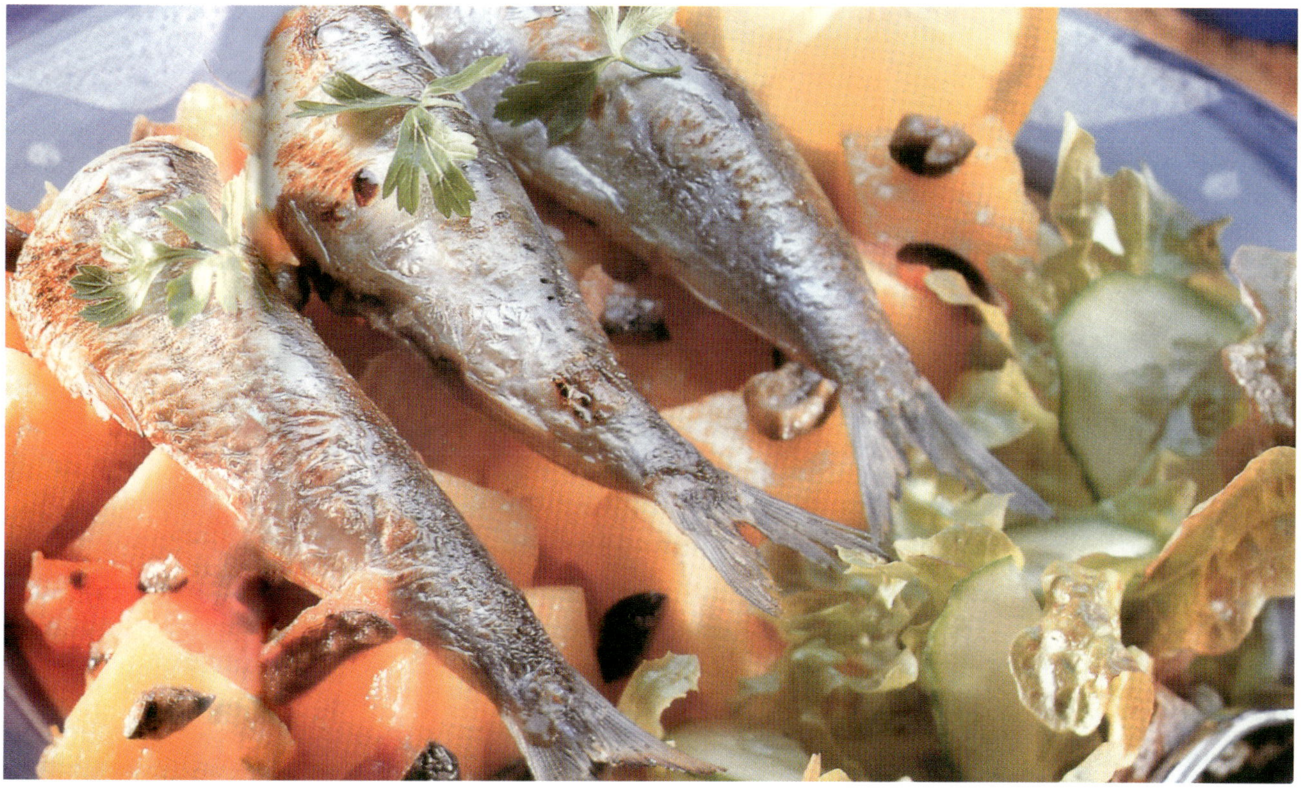

1 small spaghetti squash (weighing about 725 g), peeled, deseeded and diced
2 tbsp extra virgin olive oil
1 tsp olive oil
12 fresh sardines, scaled
2 large tomatoes, deseeded and diced
12 black olives, pitted and diced
freshly ground black pepper
green salad, to serve

1 Preheat the grill. Cook the diced squash in the oil for 3–4 minutes, stirring frequently, while grilling the sardines for 2–3 minutes on each side. Brush the fish with a little olive oil before cooking, just to stop them sticking to the grill rack or pan.

2 Toss the tomatoes and olives into the pan with the squash and just heat through. Season well, then pile the squash mixture onto warmed serving plates. Add the grilled sardines and a little green salad, and serve immediately.

NUTRITIONAL VALUES

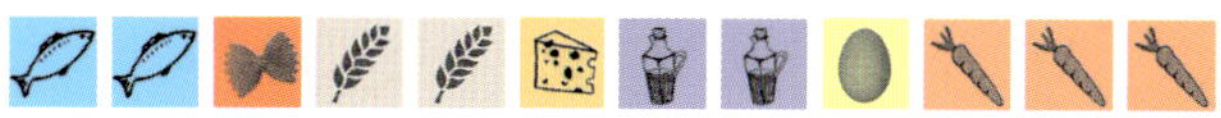

MEXICAN RICE CHICKEN

SERVES **6**

This recipe adds chicken to authentic spicy Mexican or Spanish rice.

1.5–1.75 kg chicken
2 medium onions, finely chopped
2 cloves garlic, chopped
2 serrano chillies, chopped (fresh or canned)
450 g peeled and deseeded tomatoes or
 1 can tomatoes
50 ml olive oil
450 g long-grain rice
$^1/_4$ tsp whole cumin seed
$^1/_4$ tsp saffron
900 ml chicken stock
freshly ground black pepper
200 g peas, fresh or frozen

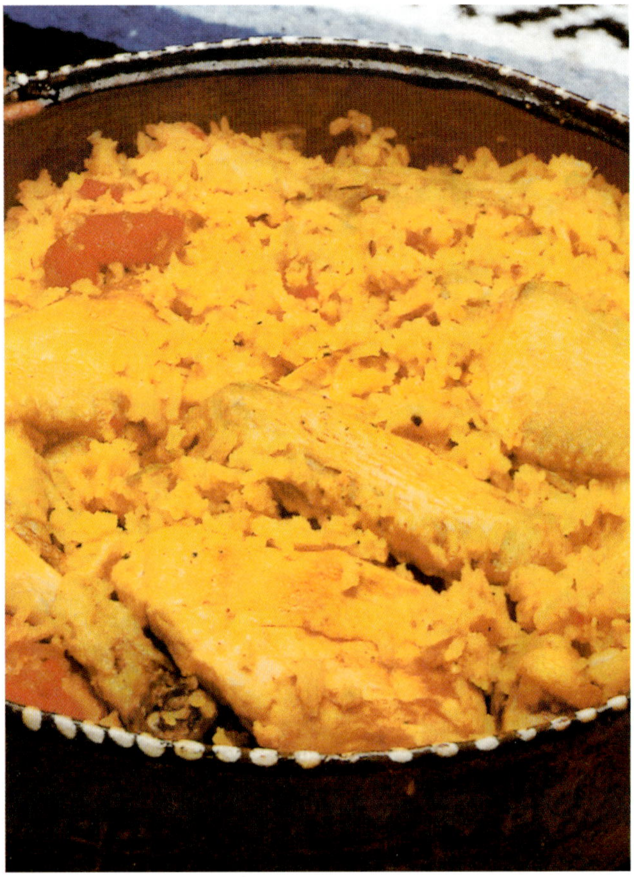

1 Cut the chicken into serving pieces. Fry until golden; drain and set aside. In the same oil, fry the chopped or sliced onion together with the garlic. Drain, and add to the chicken, together with the tomatoes, stock and spices. Bring to the boil; simmer for about half an hour.

2 Meanwhile, still in the same oil – adding a little more if necessary – fry the rice until it is golden, stirring frequently. Add the rice to the chicken; mix well; bring back to the boil, stirring frequently.

3 When the rice has absorbed all the visible liquid (10–20 minutes), add the peas; stir briefly; then cover tightly and simmer over very low heat for another 20 minutes or so.

NUTRITIONAL VALUES

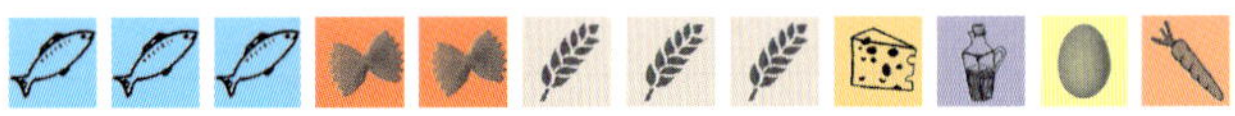

CHICKEN WITH 40 CLOVES OF GARLIC

SERVES **4**

Although 40 cloves of garlic may sound like a huge quantity, they are roasted in their skins and impart the most delicious flavour to this famous French dish from Dauphine.

large bunch of parsley, thyme and rosemary

2 bay leaves

1 whole chicken, weighing approximately 1.75 kg

salt substitute (see page 18) and freshly ground black pepper

7 tbsp olive oil

40 garlic cloves, unpeeled

90 g plain flour

5 tbsp water

GRAVY (OPTIONAL)

300 ml chicken or vegetable stock

2 tbsp cornflour

5 tbsp low-fat yoghurt

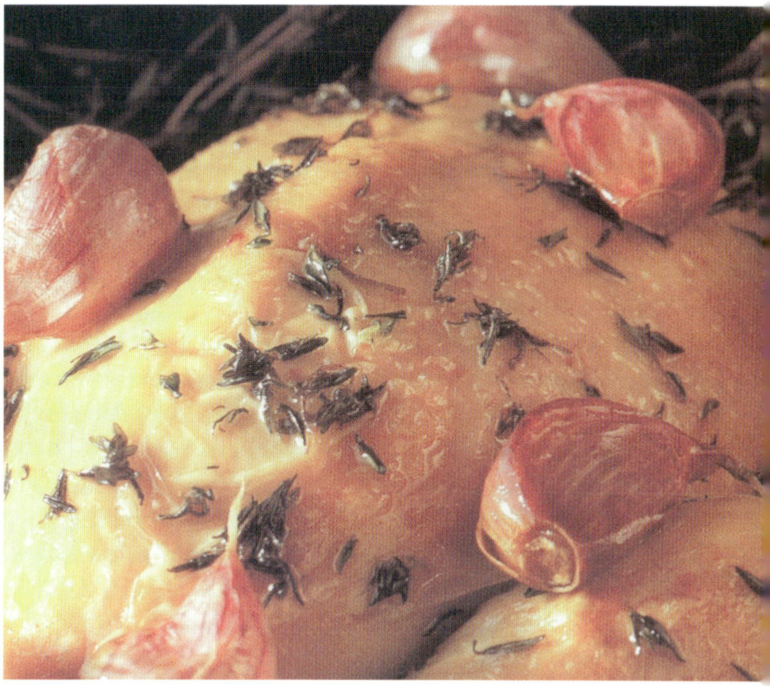

1 Preheat the oven to 180°C/gas mark 4. Form the herbs into two bouquet garnis, one slightly smaller than the other. Wash and pat dry the chicken and season inside and out with the pepper. Place the smaller bouquet garni in the cavity of the chicken. Pour the oil into a casserole which is large enough to hold the chicken with the lid on, and add the second bouquet garni and the garlic cloves. Gently heat the oil on the hob. Add the chicken and turn it to coat it in oil, ensuring the herbs remain beneath the chicken.

2 Mix the flour and water to form a thick paste. Roll the paste into a long rope shape and place this around the edge of the casserole to act as a seal for the lid. Roast in the oven for $1\frac{1}{2}$ hours. To serve, either break and clean off the seal before taking the dish to the table or break the seal in front of your guests, filling the room with a delicious aroma.

3 If you decide to make the gravy, remove the chicken to a warmed serving dish along with about two-thirds of the garlic cloves, then remove and discard the bouquet garni from the casserole. Place the casserole on the hob and heat over a medium–high heat. Squeeze the purée from the remaining garlic cloves and mix into the cooking juices. Pour in the stock and mix well. Mix the cornflour with 1–2 tablespoons of water to form a smooth paste. Add to the casserole, stirring to prevent any lumps. Once the gravy has thickened add the low-fat yoghurt. Heat through and serve with new potatoes, broccoli or green salad.

NUTRITIONAL VALUES

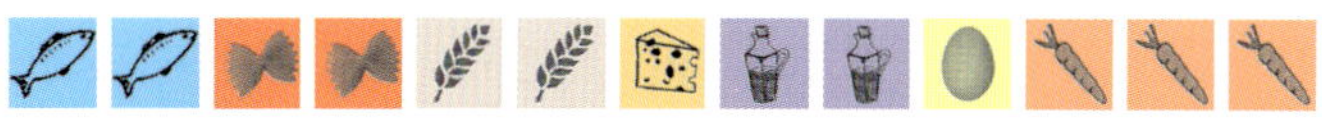

RABBIT WITH MUSTARD AND PRUNES

SERVES **4**

This risotto combines rabbit with a rich, sharp mustard and sweet juicy prunes.

450 g rabbit, diced
freshly ground black pepper
2 tbsp wholegrain mustard
8 tbsp olive oil
1.1 litres chicken stock
6 shallots, quartered
400 g arborio rice
150 ml dry white wine
1 tbsp chopped fresh thyme or 1 tsp dried
75 g no-need-to-soak dried prunes
fresh thyme, to garnish

1. Season the rabbit and coat with the mustard. Heat the oil in a large saucepan until sizzling, then fry the rabbit for 8–10 minutes all over until golden.
2. Meanwhile, pour the stock into a saucepan and bring to the boil. Reduce the heat to a gentle simmer.
3. Reduce the heat under the pan with the rabbit and gently fry the shallots for 2–3 minutes until just softened. Add the rice and cook, stirring, for 2 minutes until well coated in the rabbit juices.
4. Add the wine and thyme and cook gently, stirring, until absorbed. Ladle in the stock gradually until half is used, then add the prunes. Continue ladling in the stock until it is all absorbed and the rice is thick, creamy and tender. This will take about 25 minutes.
5. Adjust the seasoning and serve garnished with thyme.

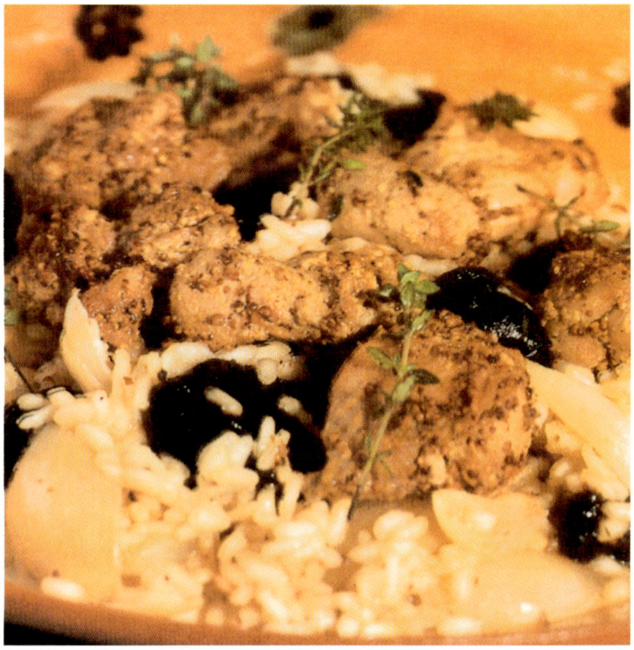

NUTRITIONAL VALUES

RABBIT STEW WITH LEEKS AND WILD MUSHROOMS

SERVES **4**

Wild mushrooms give this stew a heavenly accent. It is not a difficult dish. Start a day ahead by marinating the rabbit pieces, then use the marinade as part of the stewing liquid. The stew forms an excellent gravy.

1.5 kg rabbit, cut into 8 serving pieces
60 ml olive oil
120 ml dry white wine
2 sprigs fresh tarragon, bruised to release flavour
1 bay leaf
2 cloves garlic, finely chopped
2 carrots, peeled, and sliced
2 leeks, white part only, thinly sliced
dash of freshly ground black pepper
60–120 g flour
2 tbsp olive oil
250 ml dry white wine
475 ml chicken stock (see page 24)
2 tbsp olive oil
225 g wild mushrooms, any combination, quartered
hot noodles or cooked rice to serve

1 In a glass, or other non-reactive dish, make the marinade. Combine the olive oil, wine, tarragon, bay leaf, garlic, carrots, 1 leek and ground pepper. Marinate the rabbit for 24 hours in the refrigerator, turning and basting several times.

2 Remove the rabbit and vegetables from the marinade, and discard the bay leaf. Save the marinade. Finely chop the tarragon. Pat the rabbit pieces dry and dredge in flour.

3 In a Dutch oven or large pot, heat 2 tablespoons olive oil. Brown the rabbit pieces on all sides, then remove. Sauté the vegetables from the marinade, along with 1 fresh chopped leek. Add the tarragon, rabbit pieces, wine and stock to the pot and bring to the boil. Reduce the heat and simmer for 30 minutes, uncovered. Skim fat from surface.

4 Heat some olive oil in a small frying pan. Sauté the mushrooms for about 7 minutes. Add the mushrooms to the stew, and continue cooking until the rabbit is tender, about 30 minutes longer. Serve the stew over hot noodles or rice.

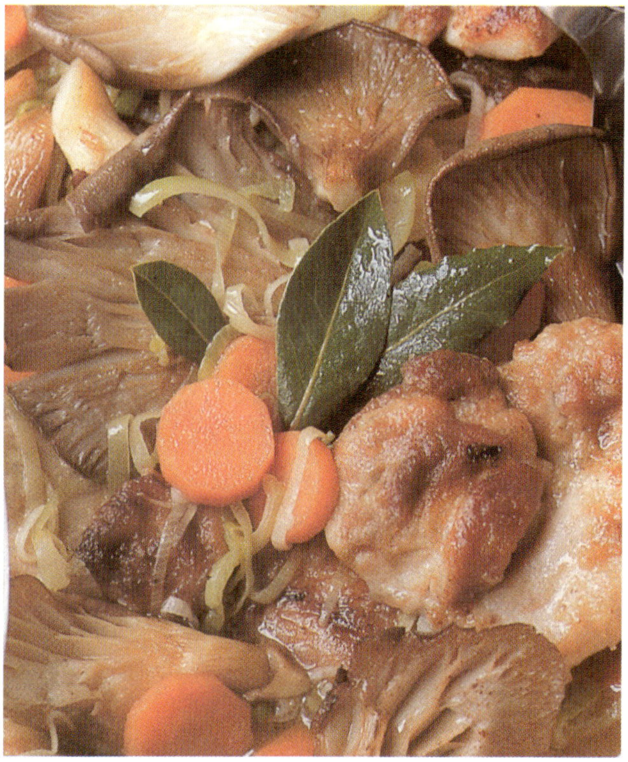

NUTRITIONAL VALUES

BRAISED WHOLE FISH IN HOT VINEGAR SAUCE

SERVES **4–6**

What better way to present a fish dish? If you're not too keen on hot sauces, then just take away some of the chillies to soften the impact.

2 slices fresh root ginger

1 whole fish, 700–900 g

freshly ground black pepper to taste

4 tbsp olive oil

SAUCE

3 slices fresh root ginger

40 g canned bamboo shoots, drained

$\frac{1}{2}$ red pepper

1 small carrot

1 green chilli

2 dried chillies

2 spring onions

2 tbsp light soy sauce

3 tbsp good stock

6 tbsp vinegar

$\frac{1}{2}$ tbsp cornflour blended with 2 tbsp water

NUTRITIONAL VALUES

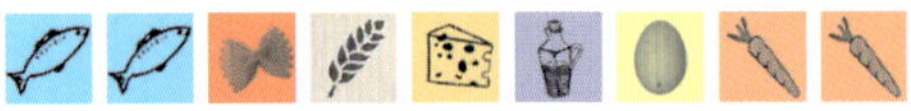

1 Finely chop the 2 slices of ginger. Clean the fish and dry well. Rub evenly inside and out with pepper, chopped ginger, and 1 tablespoon of the olive oil. Leave to season for 30 minutes. Shred the 3 slices of ginger, bamboo shoots, red pepper, carrot, chillies, discarding seeds, and spring onions.

2 Heat the remaining oil in a wok or frying pan. When hot, fry the fish for $2\frac{1}{2}$ minutes on each side. Remove and drain. Add the shredded ginger, bamboo shoots, red pepper, carrot, chillies and spring onions to the remaining oil and stir-fry over medium heat for 1 minute. Add the soy sauce, stock and half the vinegar and cook for another minute. Lay the fish back in the wok or pan and cook gently for 2 minutes on both sides, basting. Transfer the fish to a serving dish. Stir the remaining vinegar into the wok, then add the blended cornflour, stirring over high heat until the sauce thickens.

3 Pour the sauce from the wok over the length of the fish and garnish with the shredded vegetables.

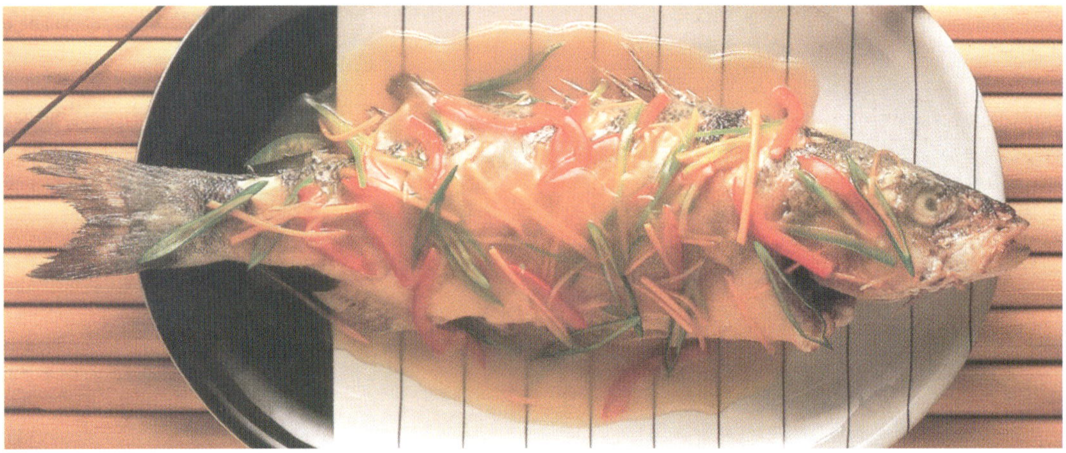

PRAWNS WITH BROCCOLI OR SPINACH

SERVES **4**

This is a lightly spiced prawn dish, which is perfectly complemented by the great texture of broccoli.

450 g broccoli or fresh spinach
2 tsp ginger and garlic paste
1 tbsp olive oil
50 g onion, finely chopped
1/4 tsp cumin seeds
2 cloves garlic, finely chopped
1/2 tsp chilli powder
1/4 tsp turmeric
1/2 tsp garam masala
3/4 tsp salt substitute (see page 18)
10 oz prawns, fresh or frozen
1 tbsp low-fat natural yoghurt
2 oz tomato, chopped

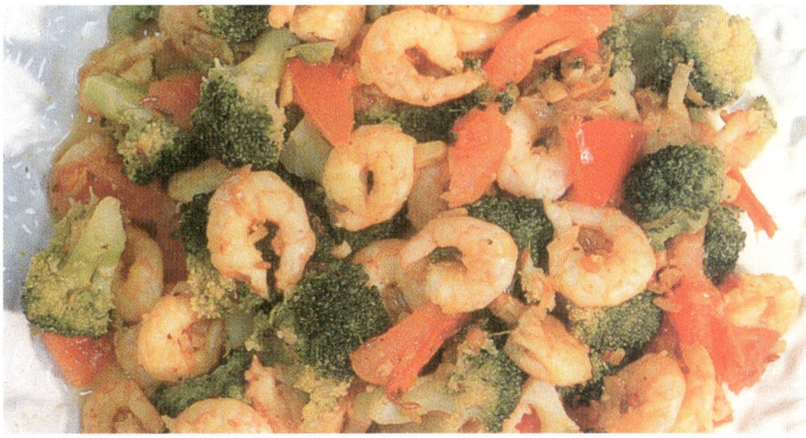

1. If using fresh prawns, wash and pat them dry.
2. Wash and chop the broccoli or spinach.
3. Put the broccoli or spinach into a medium-size saucepan and add the ginger and garlic paste, a pinch of salt substitute and 100 ml of water. Cook, uncovered, over a low heat until the broccoli or spinach is tender and almost all of the liquid has evaporated.
4. Heat the olive oil in another medium-size heavy saucepan. Fry the onion and cumin seeds until they change to a pale gold colour.
5. Add the garlic and cook for 30 seconds, than add the chilli powder, turmeric and garam masala. Cook this mixture for another minute or so, adding 1 tablespoon of water as necessary to avoid the mixture burning or sticking, and stir continuously.
6. Add the prawns and then the yoghurt. Stir-fry everything together for half a minute.
7. Add the tomato, mix it in and cook over a low heat for 2–3 minutes. Combine the cooked broccoli with the prawn mixture and cook over medium heat for another 8–10 minutes.

NUTRITIONAL VALUES

SALMON AND VEGETABLE STIR-FRY

SERVES **4**

Salmon contains a medium level of cholesterol. It is a rich source of protein, as well as vitamins A and D, and contains two fatty acids similar to those in unsaturated vegetable oils. In this recipe, a small amount of fish is combined with a contrasting mixture of fresh vegetables.

6 tbsp olive oil
$^{2}/_{3}$ cup carrots, scraped and cut into matchstick strips
2 celery sticks, thinly sliced diagonally
100 g thinly sliced broccoli spears
4 spring onions, trimmed and cut diagonally into 1.2 cm pieces
2 tbsp fresh ginger root, peeled and finely chopped
2 cloves garlic, finely chopped
175 g jar baby corn-on-the-cobs, drained
900 g tail-end salmon, skinned, boned and cut into thick strips

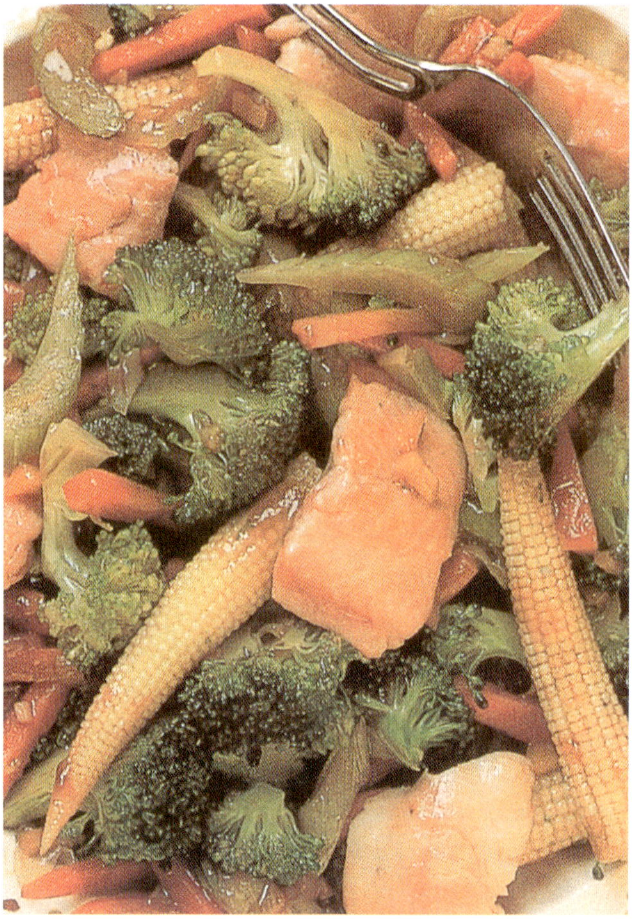

FOR THE SAUCE

1 tbsp cornflour
2 tbsp soy sauce
3 tbsp sweet sherry
2 tbsp clear honey
juice of 1 lemon
2 tbsp water

1 First make the sauce. Put the cornflour into a small bowl and stir in the soy sauce. Gradually stir in the remaining ingredients, then set aside.

2 Heat the oil in a large, shallow frying pan or a wok. When it is hot, add the carrots and celery and stir-fry for 2 minutes. Add the broccoli, onions, ginger and garlic and continue to stir-fry for 1 minute, then stir in the baby corn-on-the-cobs.

3 Pour the sauce onto the vegetables and stir for about 1 minute, until it thickens slightly.

4 Push the vegetables to the sides of the pan and add the salmon in the centre. Stir-fry for 3-4 minutes, until the fish strips turn pale pink. Serve at once, with brown rice or noodles.

NUTRITIONAL VALUES

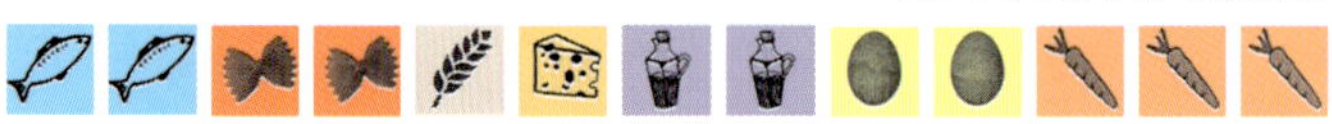

BRAISED SWORDFISH WITH PEPPERS

SERVES **4**

Red peppers are a great source of vitamin C, containing higher levels than oranges.

4 swordfish steaks (about 175 g each)
4 tbsp olive oil
4 cloves garlic
1 medium onion, roughly chopped
1 medium red pepper, deseeded and finely sliced
125 g fresh or canned plum tomatoes, roughly chopped
1 chilli pepper
84 ml dry white wine
pepper to taste

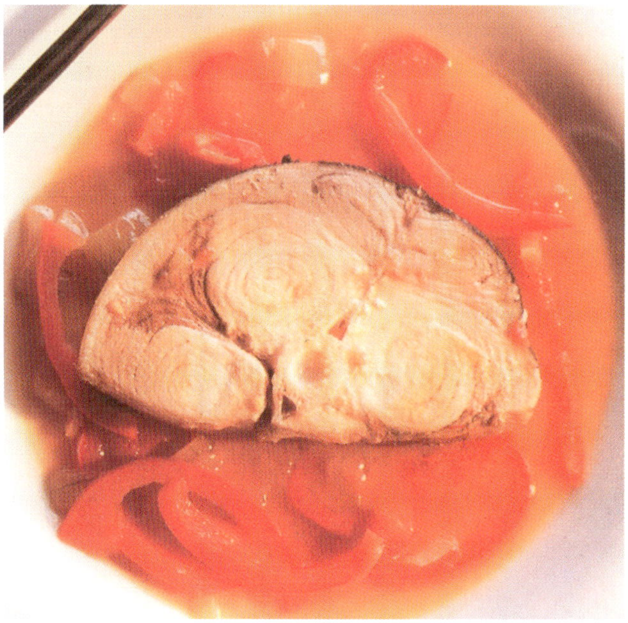

NUTRITIONAL VALUES

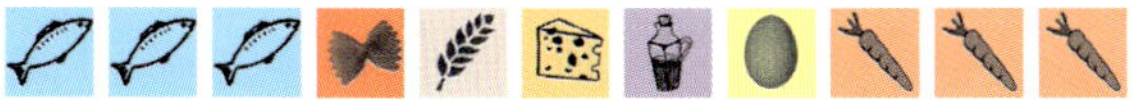

1 Wash and thoroughly dry the steaks. Heat the oil over a high heat and seal each steak on each side.

2 Remove the fish from the pan and set it aside. Turn down the heat to medium and add the whole cloves of garlic and the onions.

3 Turn the heat once more to high and cook the onions until the edges begin to catch. Reduce the flame to a gentle simmer and cook until the onions and garlic are softened.

4 When the onions are soft, add the pepper and cook until it begins to soften – about 5 minutes. Add the tomatoes, the whole chilli and the wine. Bring to a fierce boil, then add the fish. Turn the heat to a low simmer and cover the pan. Simmer until the fish is very tender, about 15 minutes.

5 Remove the fish from the pan and set it aside in a warm place. Boil up the pan juices very briskly until they are reduced to a thick, creamy mixture. Season, pour around the fish, and serve.

TOMATO AND CHICKEN CASSEROLE

SERVES **4–6**

This chicken casserole will soak up all the great flavours from the onions and garlic, to produce a lovely, succulent chicken dish.

50 ml olive oil
1.5 kg prepared chicken, cut into portions
flour, for dredging
2 large red onions, sliced
2 x 400 g cans chopped tomatoes
3 garlic cloves, crushed
freshly ground black pepper to taste
75 ml boiling water
2 tbsp red wine vinegar
chopped fresh parsley, to garnish

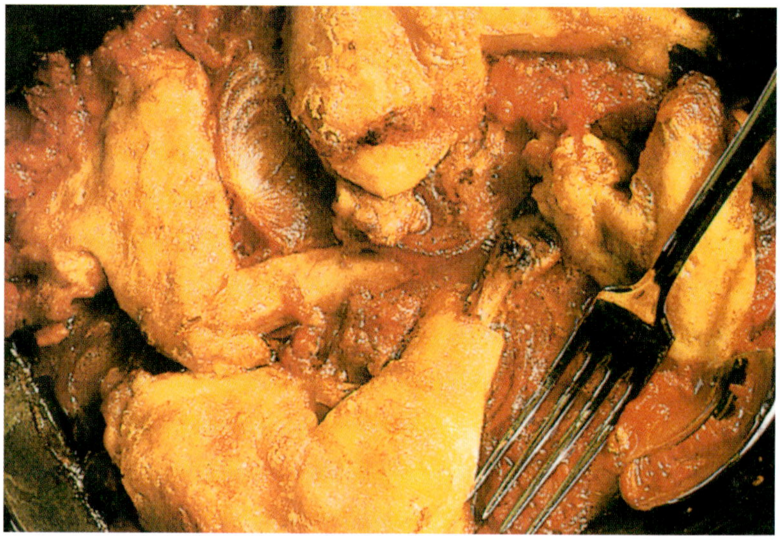

1 Preheat the oven to 190°C/gas mark 5. Heat the oil in a large, flameproof casserole. Place the chicken portions on a chopping board and dredge all over with flour. Place in the casserole and cook for about 5 minutes, or until evenly browned, turning the portions as they cook. Using a slotted spoon, transfer the chicken portions to a plate and set aside.

2 Add the onion to the casserole and cook for 3 minutes, or until softened. Return the chicken to the casserole, add the chopped tomatoes and garlic, and season with freshly ground black pepper. Add the boiling water, cover, and cook in the oven for 45–55 minutes or until the chicken is tender and the sauce has thickened.

3 In the last 5 minutes of cooking time, stir in the red wine vinegar and a little extra boiling water if necessary. Serve sprinkled with chopped fresh parsley and new potatoes or jacket potatoes.

NUTRITIONAL VALUES

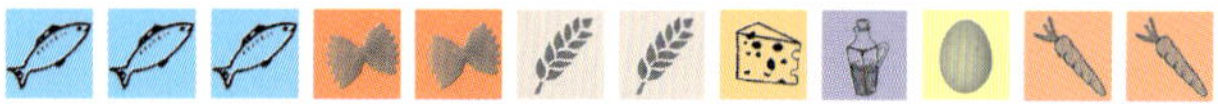

CHICKEN, MUSHROOM AND SPINACH LASAGNE

SERVES **6**

A tasty lasagne, accompanied with a crisp salad and crusty brown bread, makes for easy and informal entertaining. Prepare the lasagne in advance and chill until you are ready to cook it.

CHICKEN & NUTMEG SAUCE

8 tbsp olive oil

1 small onion, finely chopped

450 g uncooked chicken meat, cut into 1 cm cubes

125 g plain flour

900 ml semi-skimmed milk

$\frac{1}{2}$ tsp freshly grated nutmeg

freshly ground black pepper

MUSHROOM & SPINACH MIXTURE

1 tbsp olive oil

1 onion, finely chopped

3 cloves garlic, crushed

375 g flat mushrooms, finely chopped

375 g fresh spinach, washed

freshly ground black pepper

300–375 g green pre-cooked lasagne (approx. 12 sheets)

50 g Parmesan cheese, freshly grated

1. Preheat the oven to 190°C/gas mark 5

2. To make the chicken sauce, heat 1 tablespoon of the olive oil in a pan and cook the onion gently until softened. Add the diced chicken and stir-fry until the chicken is firm and cooked through.

3. In another saucepan, warm the rest of the oil. Add the flour and cook, stirring, for 1 minute. Remove from the heat and slowly blend in the milk, beating to a smooth sauce between each addition. Return to the heat and bring to the boil and cook for 1 minute. Season with the nutmeg and pepper.

4. Put one-third of the sauce into a bowl and reserve. Add the chicken and onion mixture to the remaining sauce. Place a layer of damp greaseproof paper on the surface of both sauces to prevent a skin forming.

5. For the mushroom and spinach mixture, heat the oil and cook the onion and garlic gently until softened. Add the mushrooms and cook gently for 10 minutes or until any liquid has evaporated.

6. Cook the spinach briefly in a large covered saucepan until it has wilted and reduced in volume. No need to add any water. Drain, squeeze out any excess liquid, and then chop finely. Add to the mushroom mixture and season to taste.

7. Lightly oil a deep rectangular ovenproof dish approx. 30 x 18 cm. Line the bottom and sides of the dish with some of the pasta and then layer with half the chicken sauce, pasta, spinach and mushroom sauce, more pasta, the remaining chicken sauce, pasta and the nutmeg sauce.

8. Sprinkle with the grated Parmesan and cook for 45–50 minutes or until bubbling and golden brown on top.

NUTRITIONAL VALUES

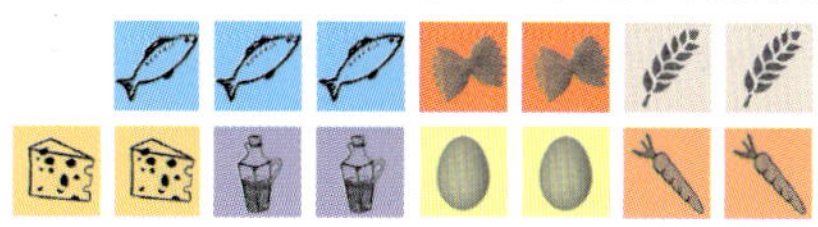

SPICED MINCED CHICKEN

SERVES **6**

The northeastern Thai version of this meat dish is characterised by the addition of uncooked sticky rice, which is first roasted (either in an oven or in a dry wok) until golden and then pounded in a mortar. It adds a slightly nutty flavour and gives the dish more body.

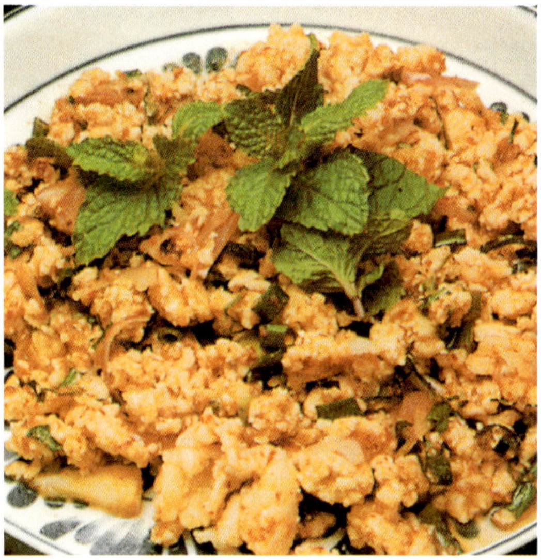

450 g finely minced chicken
25 g shallots, sliced
10 g coriander leaves
4 tbsp sticky rice, dry-fried for 8–10 minutes until brown and finely pounded
4 tbsp lemon juice, or to taste
3 tbsp fish sauce, or to taste
1 tbsp chopped dried red chilli, or to taste
fresh mint leaves, to garnish

1. Cook the chicken in a non-stick pan over low heat for 10 minutes – do not add water or oil. When cooked, transfer to a bowl and mix in well all the remaining ingredients except the mint.
2. Check the seasoning, and add more lemon juice, fish sauce or chilli if necessary. Sprinkle the mint over the top to garnish.
3. Serve accompanied by raw cabbage leaves, spring onions and raw green beans.

NUTRITIONAL VALUES

SOUTHERN STUFFED CHICKEN THIGHS

SERVES **4**

Cooking apple, walnuts, ginger, celery and liver make a tasty melange of flavours and textures. The liver is not enough to dominate the stuffing, and it is nicely complemented by the other flavours.

1 tbsp olive oil
25 g onion, chopped
25 g celery, chopped
150 g uncooked chicken livers, finely chopped
1/4 tsp ground ginger
1/4 tsp salt substitute (see page 18)
freshly ground black pepper
100–125 g soft breadcrumbs
1 green cooking apple, peeled, cored and cut into 5 mm dice
50 g walnuts, coarsely chopped
3 tbsp milk
8 chicken thighs
1/2 tsp paprika

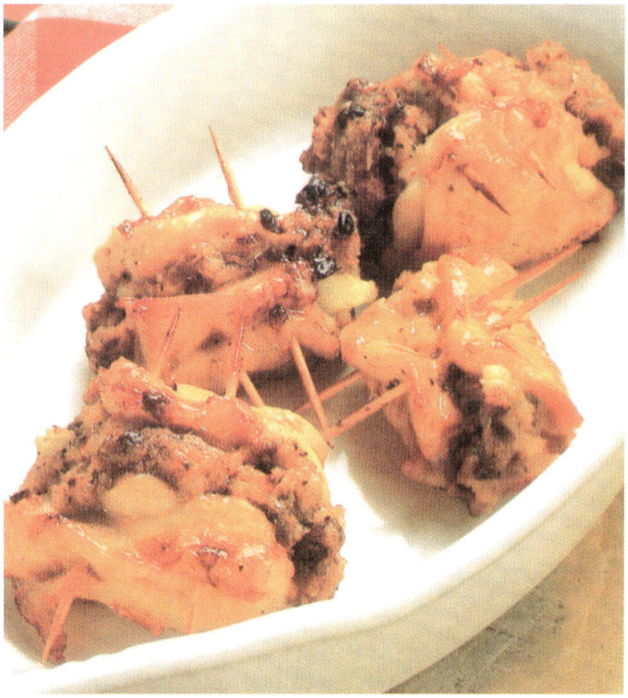

NUTRITIONAL VALUES

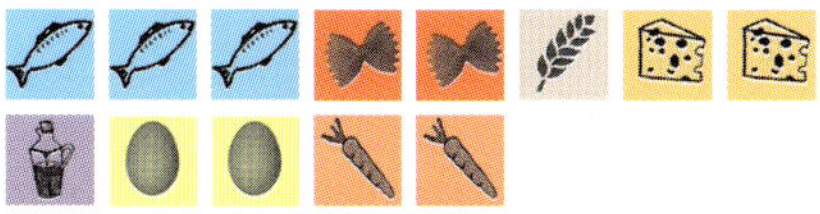

1 In a medium frying pan, sauté the onion and celery in the olive oil for 3 minutes. Add the chopped liver. Cook, stirring frequently, until the liver is thoroughly browned, about 5 minutes. Add the ginger, salt substitute and pepper, and mix well.

2 In a medium bowl, mix the breadcrumbs, apple and walnuts. Add the liver mixture. Add enough milk so that the stuffing is thoroughly moistened but not mushy.

3 Preheat the oven to 180°C/gas mark 4. Lightly grease a shallow 23 x 23 cm (or slightly larger) baking dish. Trim excess skin and fat from the chicken thighs. Remove the bone by cutting the thighs almost in half along the bone. Cut out the bone with a sharp knife. Place the boned thighs skin side down and spread out so you have a flat rectangle of meat. Place about 2 tablespoons of stuffing along the centre of each thigh. Roll up and fasten with wooden cocktail sticks or tie with string. Push any spilled stuffing back into the roll and place in baking dish, rolled edges up.

4 Brush the paprika over the thighs. Lightly sprinkle with salt substitute if desired. Bake at 180°C/gas mark 4, occasionally basting with pan juices, until the chicken is cooked through, 50–60 minutes.

BLUEBERRY GRILLED CHICKEN

SERVES **4**

Blueberries are not usually associated with grilled chicken, or grilled anything for that matter, but don't let that fool you. When you taste this chicken, you'll wonder why you haven't tried this combination sooner.

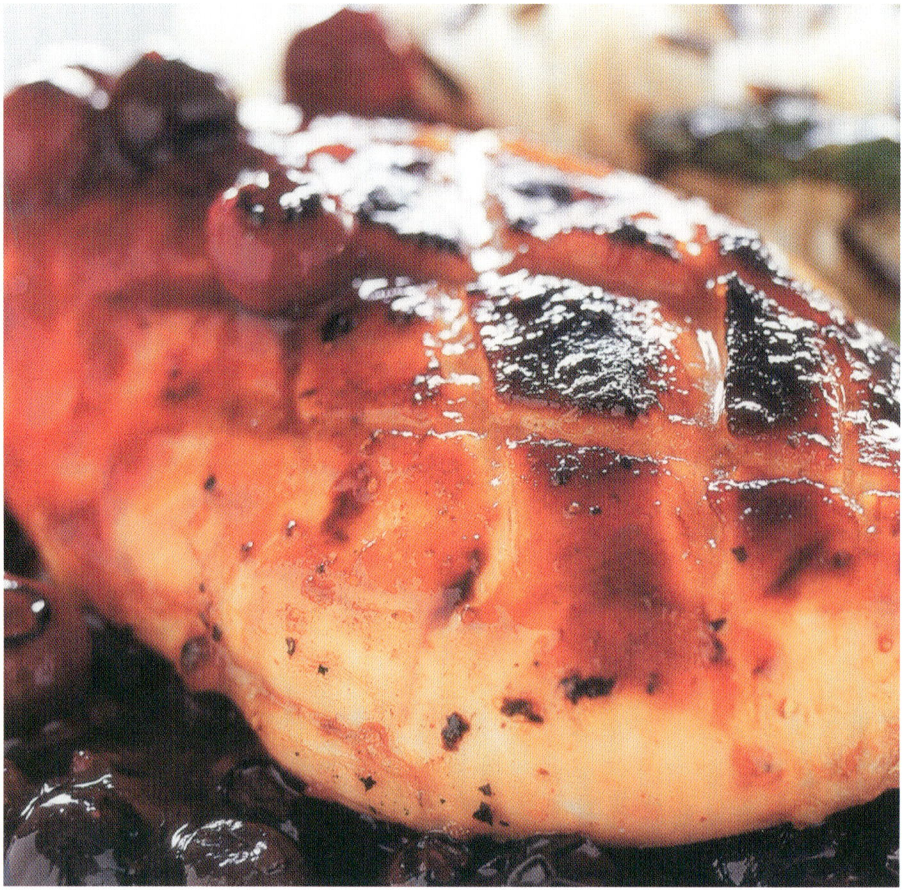

4 x 100–125 g boneless, skinless chicken breasts
125 ml apricot jam
125 ml raspberry vinegar
4 tbsp spicy brown mustard
$^1/_2$ tsp freshly ground black pepper
$^1/_4$ tsp cayenne pepper
25 g blueberries

1 Place the jam, vinegar, mustard and black pepper in a bowl and mix until well blended. Reserve 150 ml and set aside.

2 Using a sharp knife, slash criss-cross slices into the chicken flesh. Place the chicken in a glass baking dish. Pour the remaining marinade over the chicken, turning to make sure both sides are coated. Cover and leave to marinate in the refrigerator for 3–4 hours. Reserve the remaining marinade.

3 Grill the chicken over medium–hot heat, basting with the reserved marinade, 5–7 minutes per side or until the chicken is no longer pink in the middle.

4 Combine the blueberries with the 150 ml reserved marinade in a saucepan, bring to the boil and serve over the grilled chicken.

NUTRITIONAL VALUES

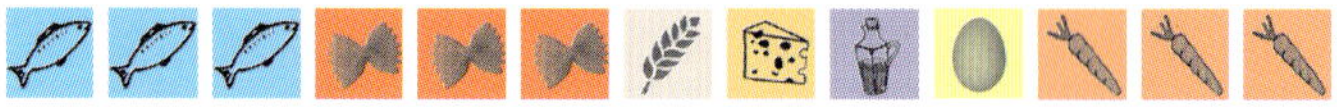

WATERCRESS SAUCE ON CHICKEN BREAST

SERVES **4**

This chicken dish looks very fresh and colourful and provides sufficient vegetables to need only the addition of new potatoes when serving.

4 part-boned chicken breasts, approx. 200 g each
50 g celery
50 g carrots, peeled
50 g green (string or snap) beans, topped and tailed
150 ml chicken stock
1 bay leaf
2 tbsp white wine
1 bunch watercress, trimmed of coarse stalks
2 spring onions, trimmed and chopped
75 g low-fat fromage frais
1 tsp cornflour, blended with 1 tsp water
freshly ground black pepper

1. Skin the chicken breasts and season lightly.
2. Prepare the vegetables and cut into julienne strips.
3. In a pan, bring the stock to a steady simmer. Add the chicken and bay leaf and cover with a tight fitting lid.
4. Cook gently for 35–40 minutes or until the chicken is tender.
5. Transfer the chicken to a warm serving plate. Add the seasoning and the spring onions to the stock. (Remove the bay leaf.) Bring to the boil and rapidly bubble until it has reduced a little.
6. Add the white wine and the watercress, reserving a few leaves for the garnish. Remove the heat and allow to stand for 1 minute for the watercress to wilt.
7. Meanwhile, cook the vegetable julienne in boiling water until tender but firm to the bite – no more than 5 minutes. Drain and keep warm.
8. Strain the stock into a measuring jug. Transfer the watercress and spring onions to a food processor or blender and add 6 tablespoons stock, the low-fat fromage frais and the blended cornflour. Purée to a smooth sauce. Season to taste.
9. Reheat gently, stirring, until thickened. Adjust the consistency of the sauce with a little more stock if desired.
10. To serve, place each chicken breast on a plate. Spoon over the vegetables julienne and pour the watercress sauce around the chicken. Garnish with the reserved watercress leaves.

NUTRITIONAL VALUES

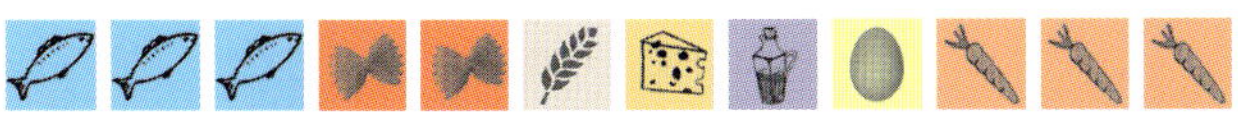

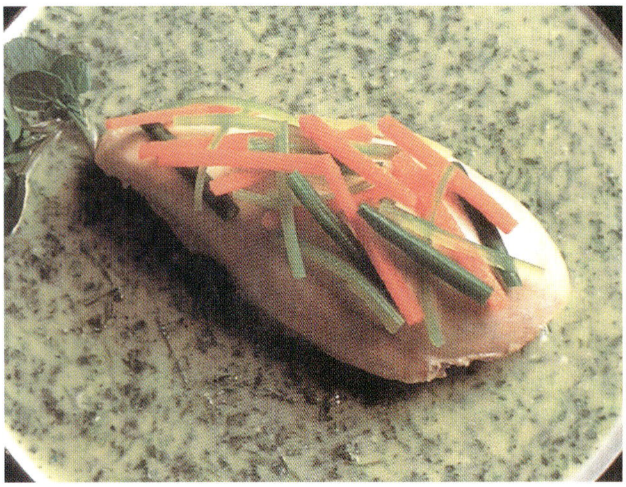

ROASTED DUCK BREASTS WITH GARLIC AND BLACK GRAPE SAUCE

SERVES **4**

Duck and fruit are natural partners. Here, duck breasts are roasted with garlic and served with a bold garlic and black grape sauce. A less fatty duck such as Barbary is good but other kinds may also be used. Served with new potatoes and green vegetables, this is an ideal dinner-party dish.

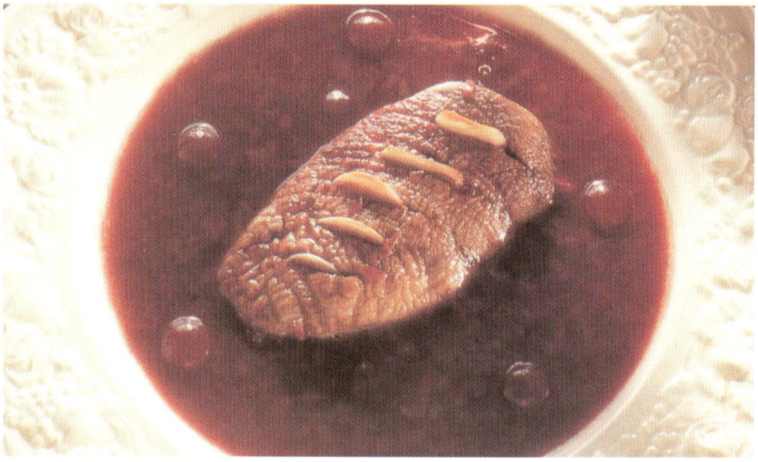

4 small–medium, skinless, boneless duck breasts

2 large garlic cloves, sliced

1 tbsp olive oil

SAUCE

2 tbsp olive oil

2 tsp sugar

2 shallots, finely chopped

2 garlic cloves, crushed

1 tsp ground nutmeg

300 ml red wine, such as claret or burgundy

180 g black grapes, halved, deseeded and skinned if the skins are tough

salt substitute (see page 18) and freshly ground black pepper

1 Preheat the oven to 200°C/gas mark 6. Take the duck breasts, cut several incisions about 1 cm deep across each breast and insert the slices of garlic. Heat up a frying pan, add the olive oil and fry the duck breasts for 4 minutes, garlic side up. Transfer to a roasting dish and roast in the oven for 15 minutes for rare meat and 20 minutes for medium-cooked meat. Once the breasts are cooked, leave them to rest in a warm place, until the sauce is ready.

2 To make the sauce, warm the oil in a small pan over high heat, add the sugar and stir until the sugar has melted. Reduce the heat to low, add the shallots, garlic and nutmeg and cook for a further 3–4 minutes. Stir in the wine, bring to the boil, reduce the heat and leave to simmer for 10–15 minutes, until the sauce has reduced by a quarter. Stir in the grapes and season. Cook for a further 2 minutes. Serve each duck breast surrounded by some of the sauce.

NUTRITIONAL VALUES

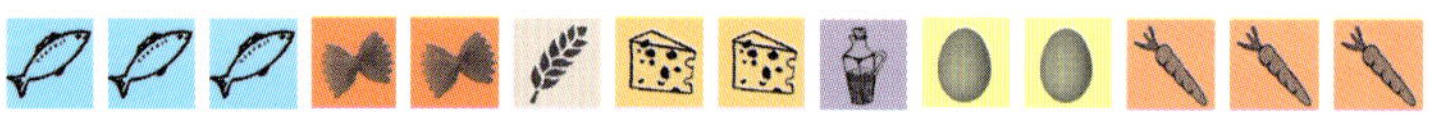

DUCK WITH PLUM STUFFING AND APPLES

SERVES **4**

This tangy mixture of rich meat and sharp fruits is ideally cooked in a claypot. Serve this dish with Chinese plum sauce, noodles and stir-fried green vegetables. This is an impressive dinner-party dish.

4 dessert apples
1 tbsp lemon juice
2 tbsp caster sugar
4 x 175 g boneless duck breasts, skinned
125 g cooked brown rice
2 medium plums, pitted and chopped
1 x 1.2 cm piece ginger root, peeled and finely chopped
1 tbsp chopped chives
freshly ground black pepper
4 tbsp dry sherry
chives and slices of plum, to garnish

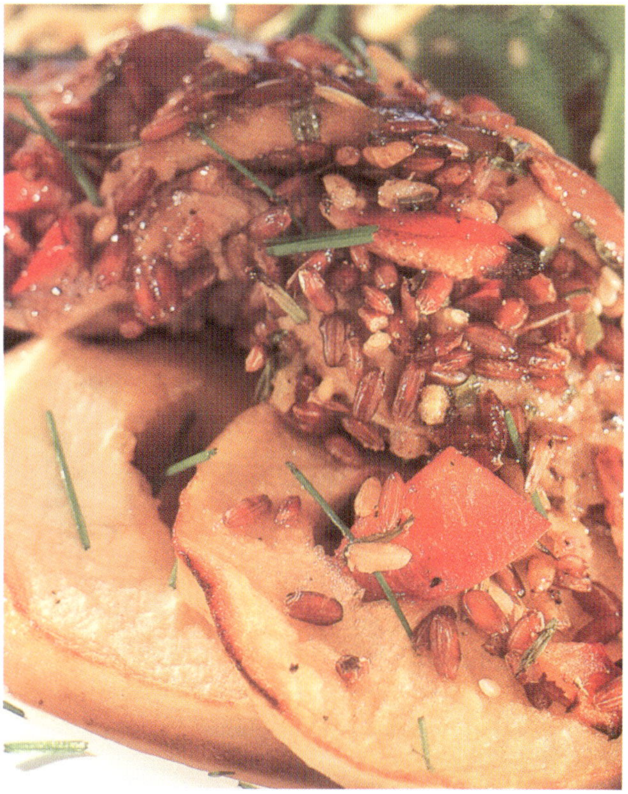

1 Pre-soak the claypot as directed. Peel, core and thickly slice the apples into rings. Place in the claypot and sprinkle with lemon juice and 4 teaspoons sugar. Set aside.

2 Wash and pat dry the duck breasts with kitchen towels. Using a small sharp knife, make a slit through the side of each, taking care not to cut through the top or bottom, to make a deep pocket in each.

3 Mix together the brown rice, plums, ginger and chives and season well. Spoon the rice stuffing into each pocket, and press together gently to seal. Secure with cocktail sticks.

4 Place the duck breasts on top of the apple rings. Spoon over the sherry and the remaining sugar and season again. Cover and place in a cold oven. Set the oven to 230°C/gas mark 8, and cook for 50 minutes. Remove the lid and cook, uncovered, for a further 15 minutes. To serve, drain the duck and arrange the apple rings on warmed serving plates. Top with a piece of duck and sprinkle with chopped chives and plum slices. Accompany with noodles and stir-fried green vegetables.

NUTRITIONAL VALUES

BRAISED PHEASANT WITH APPLE AND CREAM SAUCE

SERVES **4**

The pheasant will soak up all the goodness from the apples and cider to make a lovely, sweet-flavoured meal.

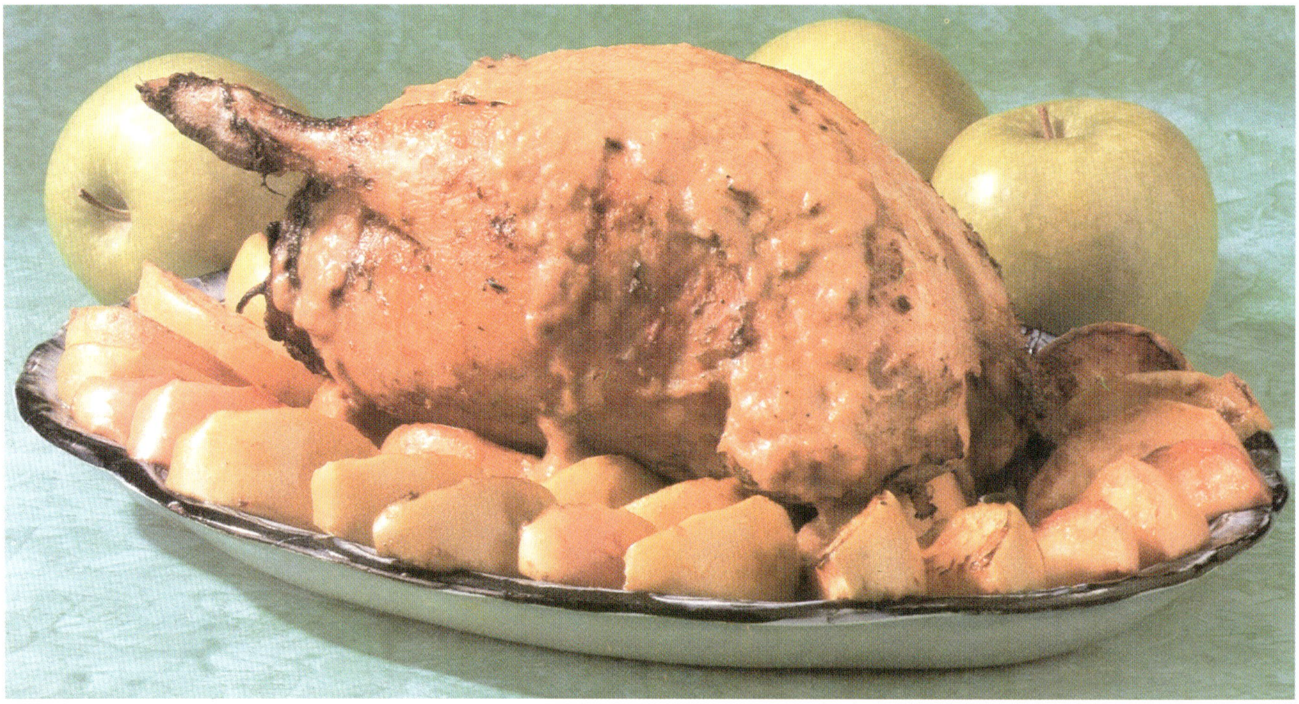

1 brace of pheasant
4 tbsp olive oil
chopped thyme, sage and rosemary
2 cooking apples
2 eating apples
300 ml cider
300 ml low-fat crème fraîche
pepper
parsley and chives to garnish

1 Brown the pheasants in some of the olive oil. Remove the pheasants. Cut them in half and rub with the chopped herbs.

2 Peel and slice the apples, and fry in the rest of the olive oil. Put the pheasants and the apples in a casserole, and pour over the cider. Cover the casserole and cook for about 40 minutes in the top of the oven.

3 Remove the pheasants from the liquid and reduce the sauce. Then add the low-fat crème fraîche and heat just to boiling point.

4 Pour over the pheasants and garnish with parsley and chives.

NUTRITIONAL VALUES

BRAISED GUINEA FOWL WITH MUSHROOMS AND BLUEBERRIES

SERVES **4**

Guinea fowl flesh is very lean and there is always the danger of its drying out, unless it is kept very moist during cooking. It is a good idea to cook it in a claypot or in a microwave or combination oven. The method given here is for a conventional oven. If you cannot find guinea fowl, wild duck or even turkey, can be substituted.

1 young guinea fowl, cut into serving pieces
2 tbsp olive oil
2 onions, sliced
2 carrots, sliced
150 g large mushrooms, sliced
4 juniper berries
150 g blueberries, fresh or frozen
2 tbsp dry red wine
375 ml chicken broth
1 bay leaf
1/2 tsp black pepper
1/2 tsp salt substitute (see page 18)
extra berries for decoration

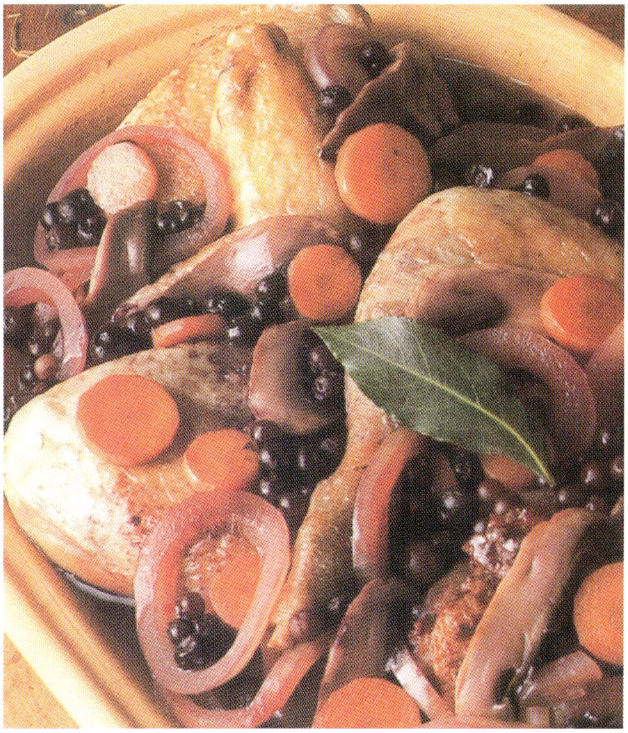

NUTRITIONAL VALUES

1 Remove all fat from the guinea fowl pieces. Pour 1 tablespoon of the olive oil into a non-stick frying pan and heat it. Quickly sauté the guinea fowl over high heat until the meat is no longer red. Transfer the meat to a casserole with a tight-fitting lid.

2 Pour the second tablespoon of olive oil into the frying pan and add the onions. Fry them until they are transparent, then add the carrots. Cook for another 5 minutes, then toss in the mushrooms. When the mushrooms start to give off their juice, transfer all the ingredients in the frying pan to the casserole and add the remaining ingredients. Cover the casserole tightly.

3 Preheat the oven to 160°C/gas mark 3. Put the casserole in the oven and cook for 2 hours. To serve, remove the guinea fowl from the casserole, drain it and season just before serving. Strain the liquid in the pan and pour a little over the meat. Serve the rest in a sauce boat.

4 Baked potatoes in their jackets or a purée of root vegetables would go well with the guinea fowl. As it will probably be served on a special occasion, a three-colour mould could be made of a layer each of boiled and puréed yellow turnips, of puréed green peas and of yams or parsnips. It can be simmered in a water bath in the oven for the last hour of cooking and un-moulded just before serving.

PHEASANT WITH CRANBERRIES

SERVES **4**

Cranberries add a tartness to any dish and they are a perfect foil for game. The mixture of sweet spices and fruit in this recipe makes this a particularly good choice for a Christmas meal, but can be enjoyed all year round.

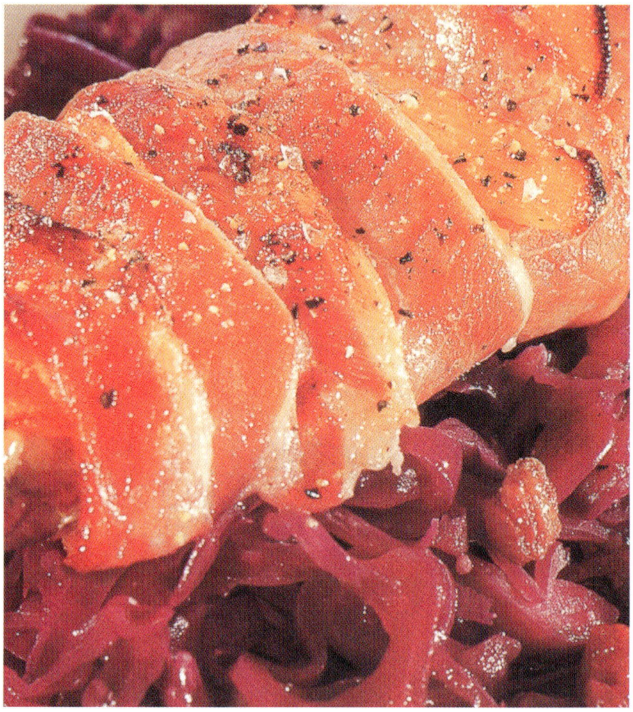

450 g red cabbage, shredded
1 large red onion, peeled and shredded
2 tbsp red wine vinegar
40 g golden raisins
150 g cranberries, thawed if frozen
50 g light brown sugar
1 cinnamon stick, broken
6 whole cloves
6 cardamom pods, split
250 ml dry red wine
4 x 150 g boneless pheasant breasts, skinned
freshly ground black pepper
4 slices lean bacon, trimmed
1 small orange
wedges of orange and fresh herbs, to garnish

1 Presoak the claypot as directed. Place the red cabbage and onion in the base of the pot and mix in the vinegar to coat. Add the raisins, cranberries, sugar and spices. Mix well. Pour over the red wine and set aside.

2 Wash and pat dry the pheasant breasts with kitchen towels. Season on both sides. Cut the lean bacon into thin lengthways strips and wrap around each breast.

3 Using a vegetable peeler, pare off 4 pieces of orange rind and carefully tuck a piece under the bacon.

4 Place the pheasant breasts on top of the cabbage mixture. Extract the orange juice and spoon over the pheasant. Cover and place in a cold oven. Set the oven to 220°C/gas mark 7, and cook for 1 hour until tender and done.

5 Remove the pheasant breasts and discard the orange rind if preferred. Drain the cabbage and discard the spices. Pile onto warmed serving plates and top each with a pheasant breast. Garnish and serve with green vegetables and cranberry sauce.

NUTRITIONAL VALUES

PORK AND CABBAGE COBBLER

SERVES **4**

A cobbler has a biscuit topping. Here the mixture of pork, red cabbage and apple is turned into a hearty meal by adding a crown of savoury biscuits.

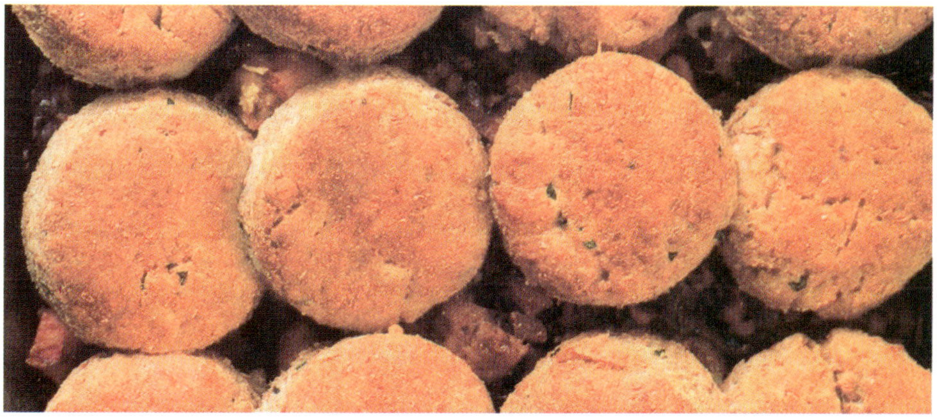

- 1 tbsp olive oil
- 450 g lean minced pork
- 1 large onion, chopped
- 1 garlic clove, crushed (optional)
- 1 tbsp fennel seeds (optional)
- 2 tbsp plain flour
- 2 dessert apples, peeled, cored and chopped
- 375 ml chicken or vegetable stock
- 675 g red cabbage, shredded
- freshly ground black pepper

TOPPING

- 250 g wholemeal flour
- 3 tsp baking powder
- 1/4 cup butter
- 3 tbsp grated Parmesan cheese
- 125 g grated Cheddar cheese
- 2 tbsp chopped fresh parsley
- 170 ml milk plus extra for glazing

1. Heat the oil, add the pork and stir over medium heat until lightly browned. If the meat yields a lot of fat, pour some off at this stage, then add the onion, garlic and fennel (if used). Cook, stirring, for 10 minutes to soften the onion slightly before stirring in the flour, apples and stock.
2. Bring to the boil, stir in the cabbage and pepper, then simmer for 10 minutes. Transfer the mixture to a baking dish.
3. Preheat the oven to 220°C/gas mark 7.
4. For the topping, mix the flour and baking powder in a bowl, then cut in the butter. Add some seasoning, then stir in the Parmesan, Cheddar and parsley. Mix in enough milk to bind the ingredients in a soft dough. Turn the dough out on a lightly floured surface, and roll it out to about 2.5 cm thick. Cut out 12 small round biscuits, re-rolling the trimmings as necessary.
5. Overlap the biscuits on top of the pork mixture, then brush them with a little milk. Bake for 20–25 minutes, until the biscuit topping is well risen and golden brown. Serve freshly baked.

NUTRITIONAL VALUES

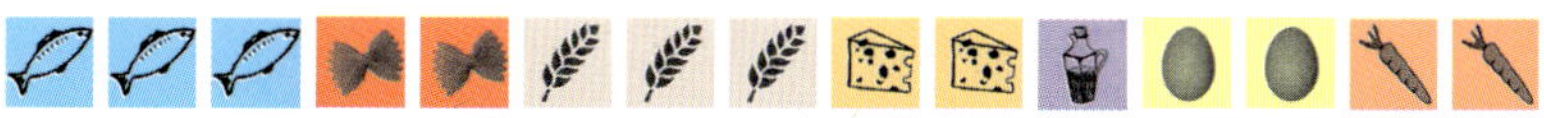

BEEF AND VEGETABLE HOTPOT

SERVES **4–6**

A wide variety of ingredients can be added to this dish. Traditionally it is prepared over a burner at the table.

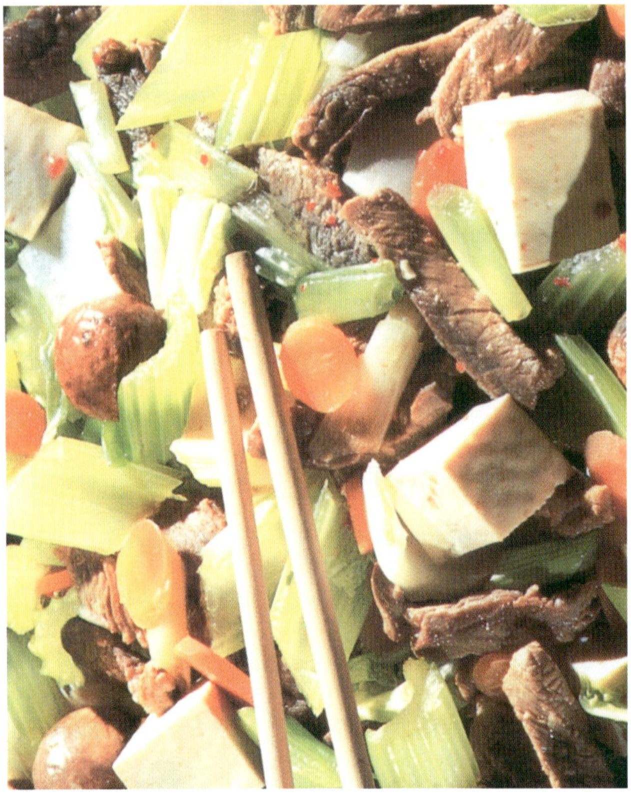

550 g sirloin or fillet of beef, partly frozen

725 ml brown veal or chicken stock

6 celery sticks, cut into 5 cm pieces

2 young carrots, finely sliced diagonally

8 chestnut mushrooms

8 spring onions, cut diagonally into 5 cm pieces

6 Chinese leaves, cut into 5 cm pieces

$1\frac{1}{2}$ cakes of bean curd, cut into 2.5 cm cubes

MARINADE

2 tsp sesame seeds

40 g sugar

1 fresh red chilli, deseeded and finely chopped

6 tablespoons soy sauce

1 plump garlic clove, finely crushed

1 For the marinade, heat a dry heavy-based saucepan, add the sesame seeds, and toast until pale brown. Remove and crush finely. Mix with the remaining marinade ingredients.

2 Slice the beef and cut into 2.5 x 5 cm strips. Put into a bowl, pour over the marinade and stir to coat. Leave for 1 hour.

3 Heat a dry heavy-based pan. Remove the beef from the marinade and add to the pan. Cook briefly and quickly to sear the meat. Remove. Add the stock and any remaining marinade to the pan and bring to the boil. If using a fondue pot, boil the stock in a saucepan then pour into the fondue pot.

4 Add the celery and carrots to the pot, boil for 5 minutes, than add the mushrooms, spring onions, Chinese leaves, bean curd and beef. Cook together for 2–3 minutes then lower the heat so the stock gently simmers.

NUTRITIONAL VALUES

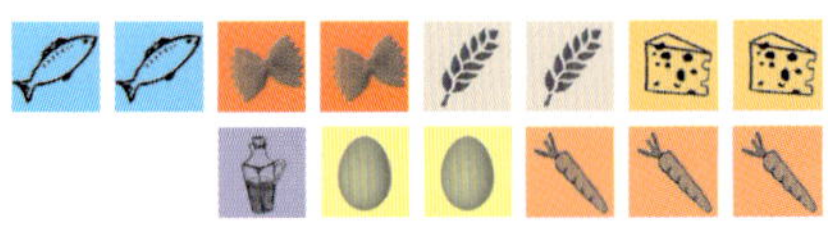

DESSERTS

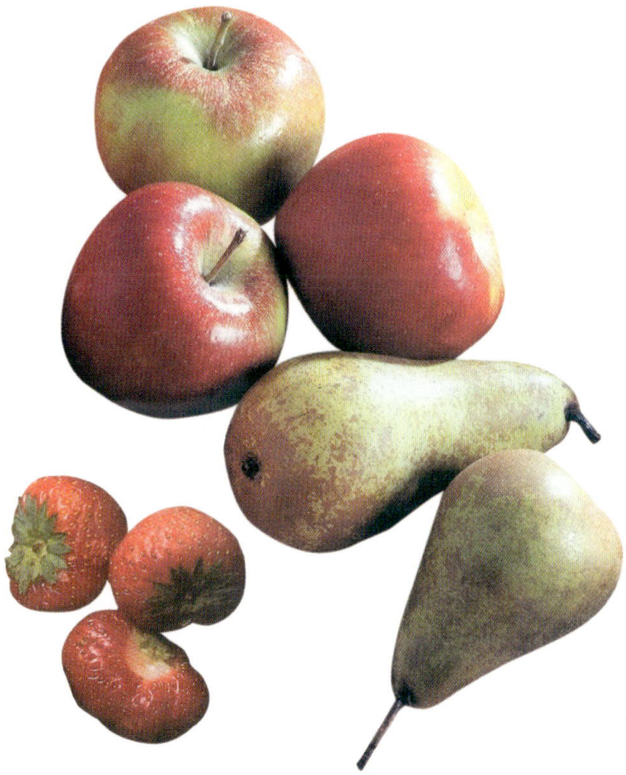

SUNSET APPLES

SERVES **4**

In a slow cooker, it is important to use firm apples. You need a variety that does not break down and become fluffy during cooking; otherwise, you will find that the apples will collapse when cooking.

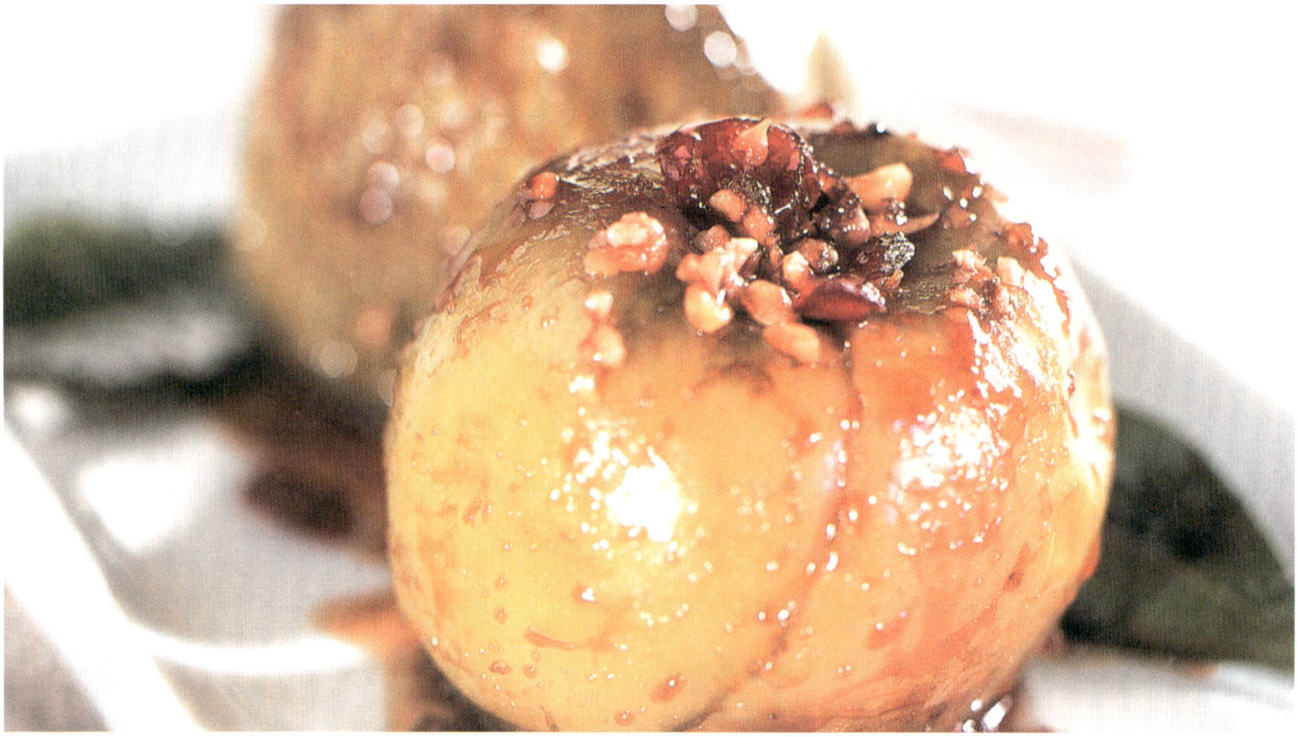

2 tbsp olive oil
4 large evenly-shaped cooking apples
25 g dried cranberries
25 g hazelnuts, chopped
3 tbsp light soft brown sugar
3 tbsp redcurrant jelly or seedless raspberry jam
4 fresh bay leaves, to garnish
low-fat crème fraîche, to serve

1 Pre-heat the cooker on high. Lightly smear the cooking pot with a little of the oil. Core the apples and rinse. Mix together the cranberries, hazelnuts and sugar and use this mixture to fill the centre of each apple. Place in the cooking pot and dot with the remaining oil.

2 Heat the jelly or jam with 3 tablespoons of water, stir until smooth, then pour over the apples. Cover and cook on low for 2–4 hours. Serve garnished with the bay leaves and with low-fat crème fraîche.

NUTRITIONAL VALUES

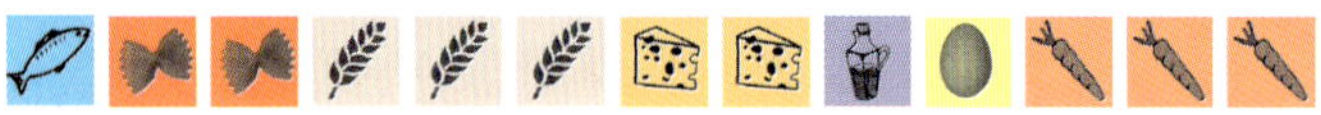

BLACKBERRY AND WHISKY OATIE

SERVES **4**

This refreshing dessert is perfect for a hot summer's day.

75 g rolled oats
5 tbsp Scotch whisky
3 tbsp clear honey
250 g low-fat cottage cheese, sieved
220 g plain low-fat yoghurt
1 tsp grated orange rind
220 g blackberries, hulled
fresh mint for decoration

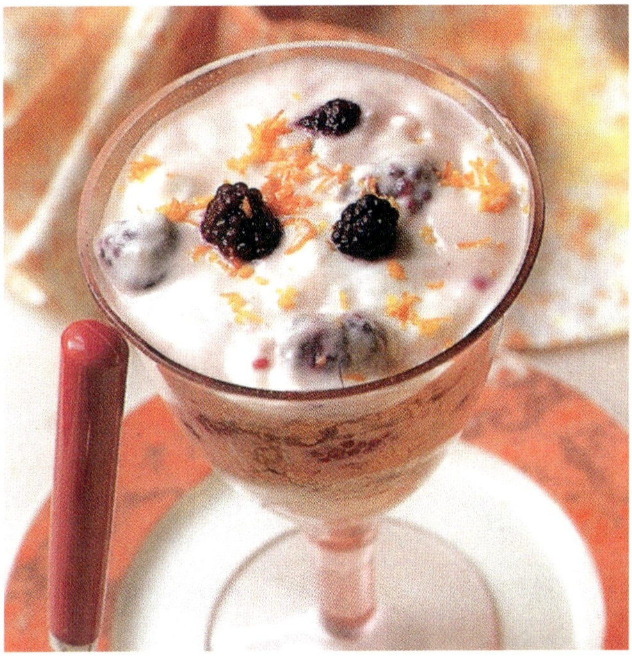

1 Put the oats and whisky into a bowl, cover, and set aside for at least 2 hours, or overnight if it is more convenient.

2 Beat together the honey, cheese and yoghurt and stir in the orange rind. Stir in most of the blackberries.

3 In 4 tall glass dessert dishes, make layers of the fruit mixture and oats, beginning and ending with the fruit. Decorate each glass with a few reserved berries and a spring of fresh mint. Serve chilled.

NUTRITIONAL VALUES

FRUDITÉES

SERVES **4**

A sweet variation of 'cruditées', this recipe is simple and easy to eat. An informal dessert to be shared with friends.

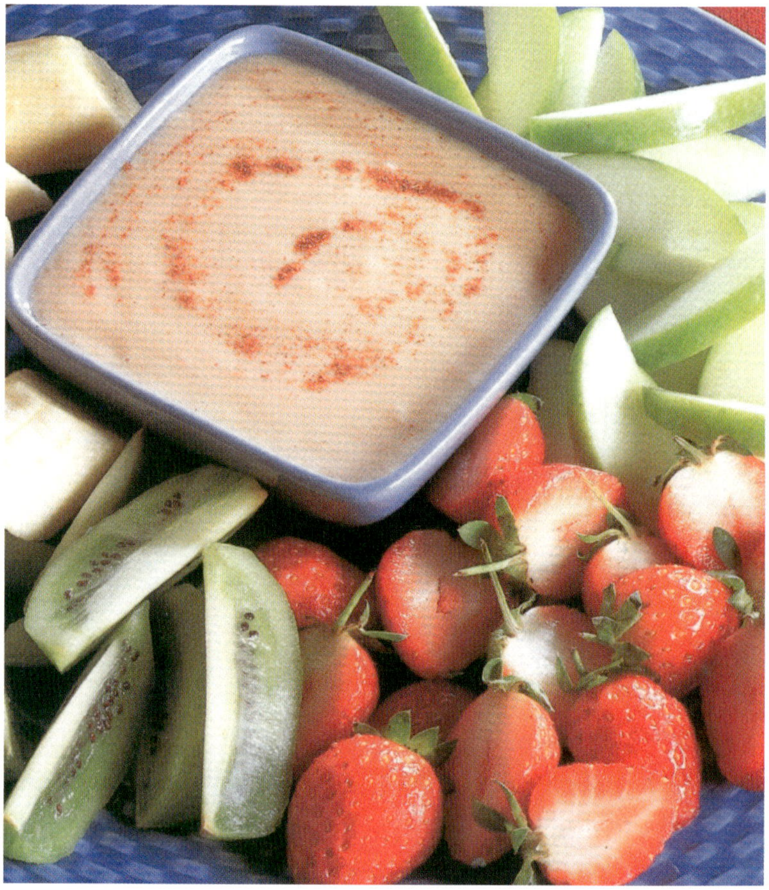

150 strawberries, halved

1 green eating apple, cored, and sliced

2 bananas, cut into 2.5 cm chunks

1 kiwi fruit, cut into 8

2 tsp lemon juice

fresh mint to decorate

FOR THE YOGHURT DIP

250 ml low-fat natural yogurt

1 tbsp soft brown sugar

dash of ground cinnamon

1 small papaya, deseeded and diced

mint and cinnamon to decorate

1 Prepare all the fruits. Sprinkle the apple and banana with the lemon juice.

NUTRITIONAL VALUES

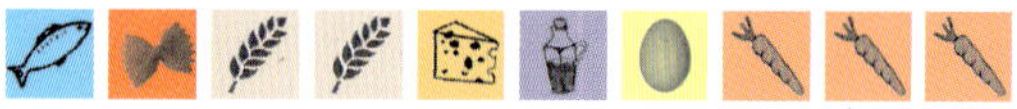

2 Place the yoghurt dip ingredients in a food processor and liquidize for 30 seconds until smooth. Spoon into a serving bowl. Place the dip on a large serving plate, sprinkle with cinnamon, and arrange the fruit around. Serve with springs of mint.

APPLE, PEAR AND CINNAMON RISOTTO

SERVES **4**

This is a real orchard dessert, delicately flavoured with cinnamon to bring out the best in the fruits.

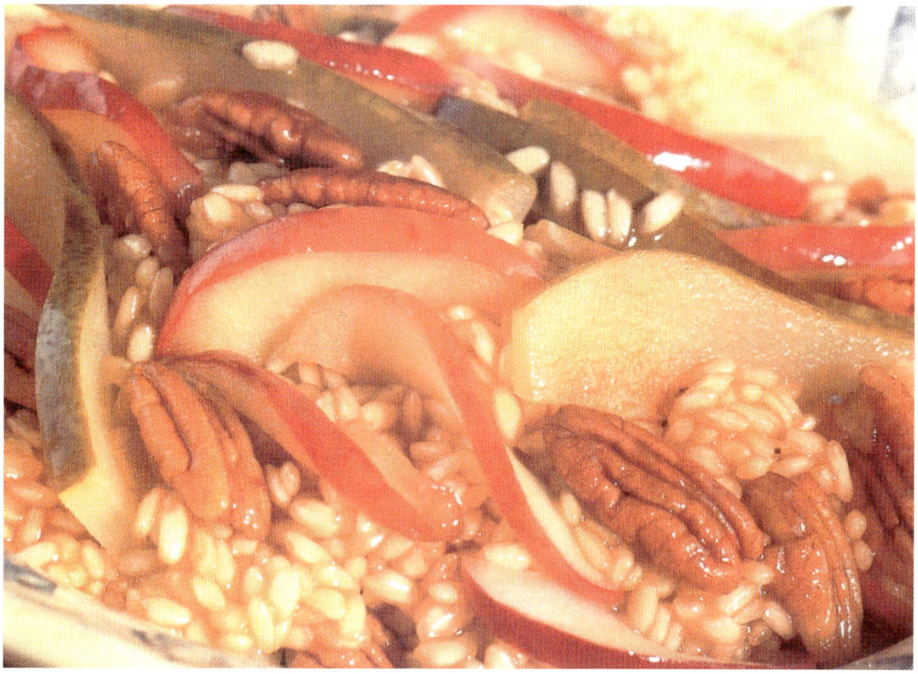

1.1 litres apple juice
4 tbsp olive oil
2 tsp ground cinnamon
25 g brown sugar
400 g arborio rice
2 red dessert apples, cored and sliced
2 dessert pears, cored and sliced
25 g pecan halves

NUTRITIONAL VALUES

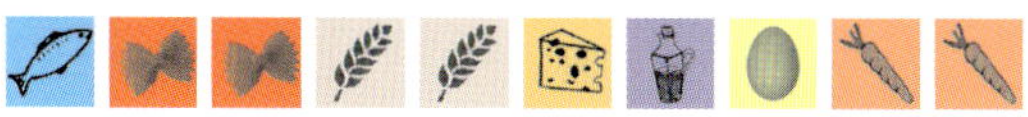

1 Pour the apple juice into a saucepan and bring to the boil. Reduce the heat to a gentle simmer.

2 Meanwhile, heat half of the oil in a large frying pan and add the cinnamon, sugar and rice. Cook gently, stirring, for 2 minutes until the rice is well coated in oil.

3 Add a ladleful of apple juice and gently cook, stirring, until absorbed. Continue adding apple juice in small quantities until the risotto is thick but not sticky, about 25 minutes.

4 Meanwhile, heat the remaining oil in a separate frying pan and cook the apples, pears and pecans for 3–4 minutes, stirring. Add the contents of the pan to the rice, mix gently and serve.

SWEET BEAN AND APPLE CRUMBLE

SERVES **6**

Adzuki beans have a slightly sweet flavour and are used in both savoury and sweet dishes. The Chinese have been making sweet bean puddings for centuries.

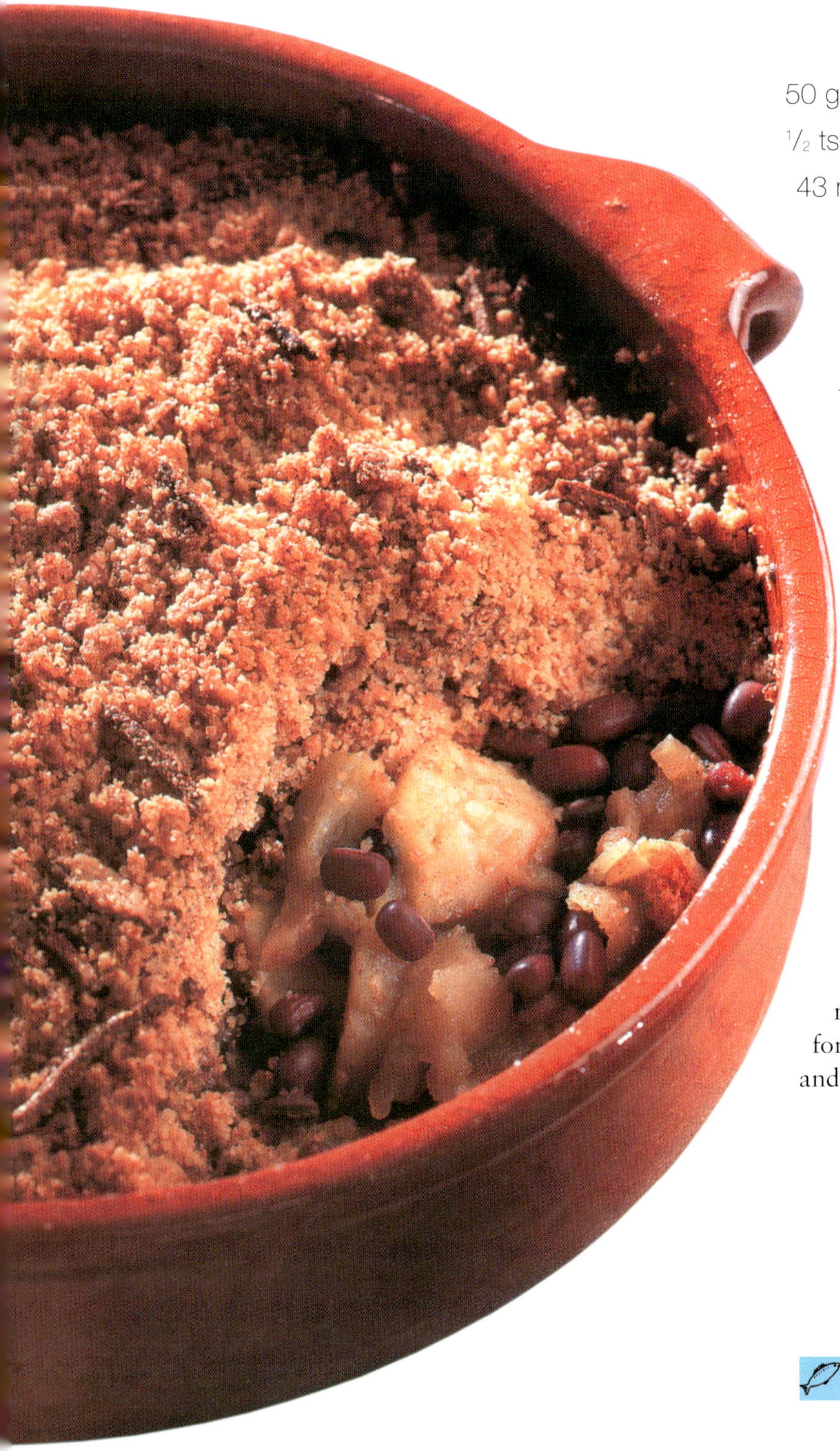

50 g adzuki beans, soaked overnight

½ tsp ground cinnamon

43 ml honey

225 g cooking apples, finely sliced

CRUMBLE

75 g butter

175 g wholemeal flour

40 g All-Bran cereal

1 tbsp light muscovado sugar

1 Drain the adzuki beans, then rinse them under cold running water. Bring to the boil in a pan of fresh water, then cover and simmer for 30 minutes or until tender. Drain and set to one side.

2 Preheat the oven to 190°C/gas mark 5.

3 Combine the cinnamon and honey and mix into the apples and adzuki beans in a suitable ovenproof dish. Blend the butter into the flour, All-Bran and sugar, then spoon the crumble mixture over the fruit. Bake in the preheated oven for 30–35 minutes, until the crumble has browned and set. Serve with low-fat yoghurt.

NUTRITIONAL VALUES

BLUEBERRY PIE

SERVES **6**

This traditional pie is high in antioxidants and is delicious served with low-fat yoghurt.

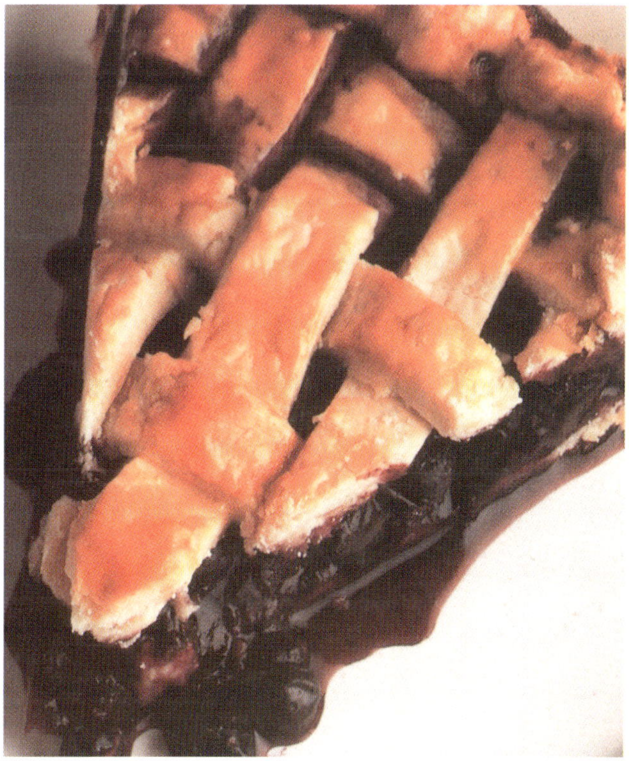

250 g cold unsalted butter, cut into small pieces
280 g plain flour
150 g caster sugar
4–5 tbsp ice water
300 g fresh blueberries
1 egg
2 tbsp water

1 Mix the butter, flour and half the sugar with a fork or fingers until the mixture has the consistency of coarse cornmeal. Add the ice water, 1 tablespoon at a time, until the dough binds.

2 Divide the dough in half, wrap in plastic, and refrigerate for about 2 hours.

3 Preheat the oven to 180°C/gas mark 4.

4 On a clean, dry surface, sprinkle some flour and roll out one of the dough pieces. Press into a 20 cm pie plate or flan tin.

5 In a medium-size bowl, toss the blueberries with the remaining sugar. Turn the blueberries into the pastry shell.

6 Roll out the remaining dough, and cut into 2 cm wide strips. Arrange on top of the pie in a criss-cross pattern. Crimp the edges.

7 Beat the egg with the water and brush over the pastry strips and edge of the shell.

8 Bake for 45–50 minutes, or until golden brown.

NUTRITIONAL VALUES

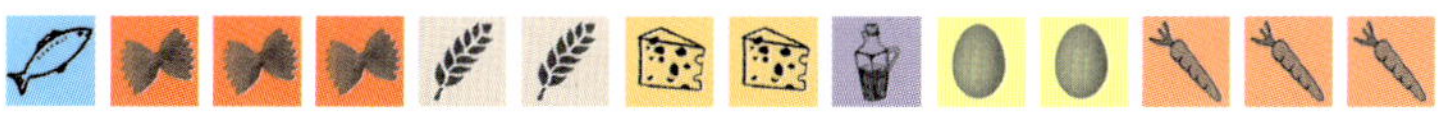

BLACKCURRANT SORBET

SERVES **4**

This delicious sorbet makes great use of the wonderful taste of blackcurrants. While frozen blackcurrants will do, try to use fresh if at all possible.

450 g blackcurrants, fresh or frozen

4 tbsp clear honey

100 g sugar

150 ml water

2 egg whites

mint sprigs for decoration (optional)

NUTRITIONAL VALUES

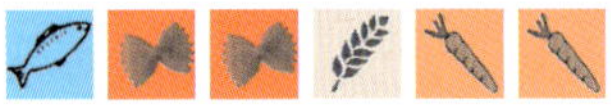

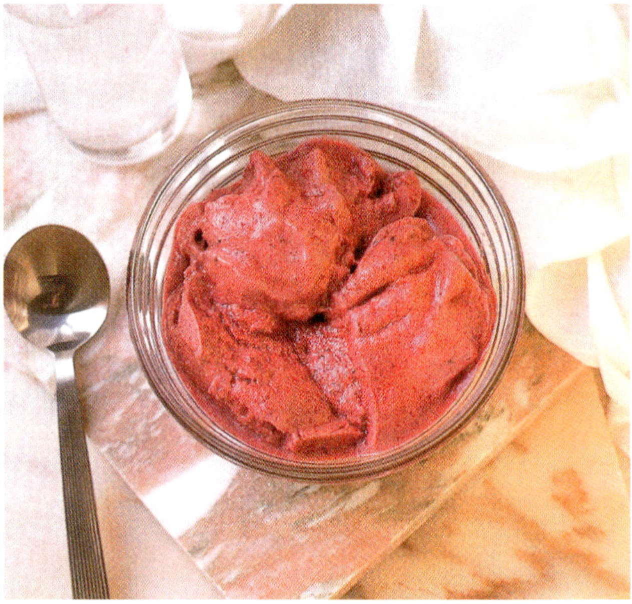

1 Put the blackcurrants, honey, sugar and water into a saucepan and bring slowly to the boil, stirring occasionally. Simmer for 15 minutes, or until the fruit is soft. Allow to cool.

2 Rub the fruit and juice through a sieve and place it in a metal ice-cube tray or a plastic freezer box. Cover with foil or a lid and freeze for 1–2 hours, until the mixture is mushy and starting to set on the outside.

3 Beat the egg whites until stiff. Turn the fruit purée out into a chilled bowl and fold in the egg whites.

4 Return the mixture to the container, cover and freeze for a further 2 hours, or until firm. Stir it once or twice during this time.

5 To serve, allow the sorbet to soften a little in the refrigerator for about 30 minutes. Spoon or scoop it into 4 individual serving glasses and top each one with a mint sprig if you wish.

DANISH APPLE CAKE

SERVES **4–6**

A lovely way to enjoy a hot summer evening. The apples are refreshing to taste and complemented by the great texture of the breadcrumb mixture.

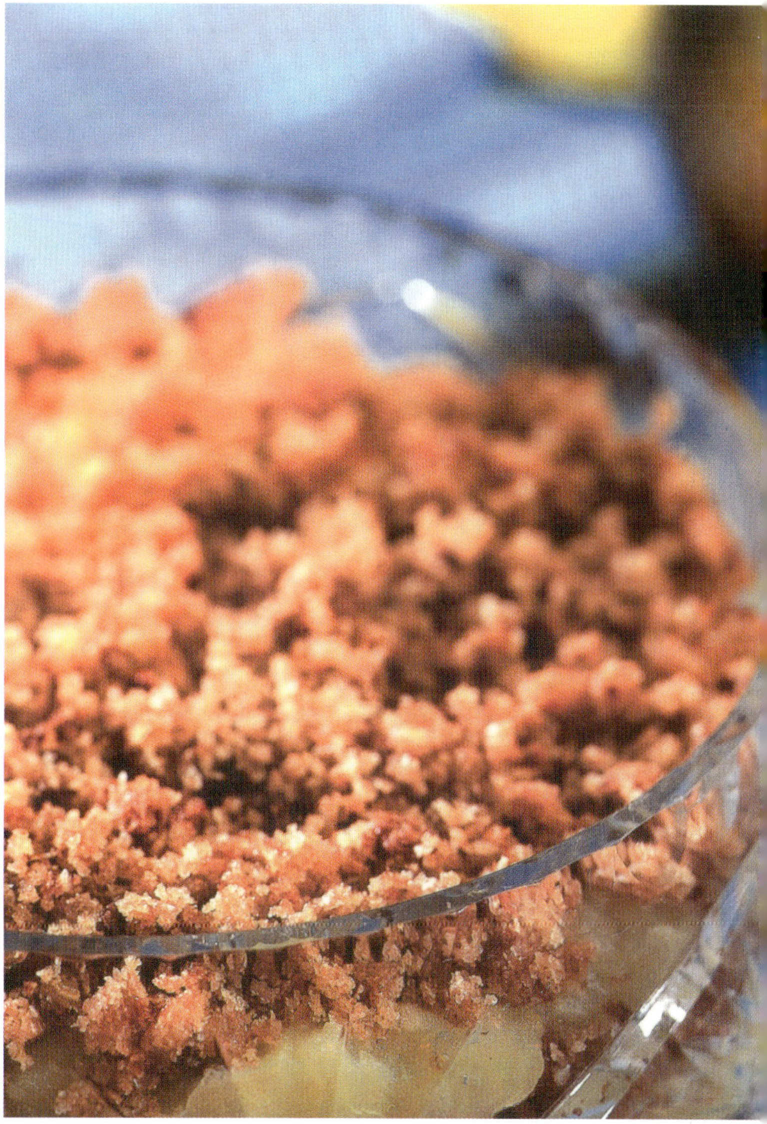

375 g fresh wholemeal breadcrumbs
34 g raw brown sugar
$5\frac{1}{2}$ tbsp unsalted butter
450 g prepared cooking apples, peeled, cored and sliced
grated rind and juice of 1 lemon

1. Mix the breadcrumbs with the sugar.
2. Melt the butter in a large frying pan, add the crumb mixture, and fry quickly until the crumbs are crisp. Set aside until needed.
3. Cook the apples with the lemon rind and juice and as little water as possible until soft. Allow to cool.
4. Turn half the apples into a glass dish, then make a layer of half the crumbs over the apples. Repeat the layers, finishing with the remaining crumbs. Let cool completely, then chill for at least 1 hour before serving.

NUTRITIONAL VALUES

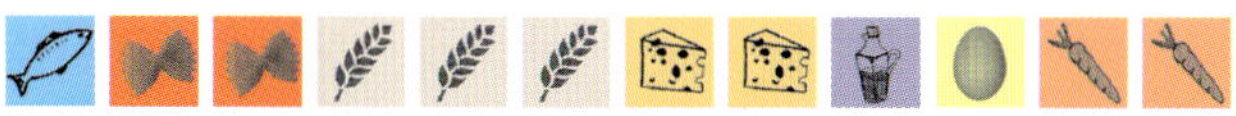

INDEX

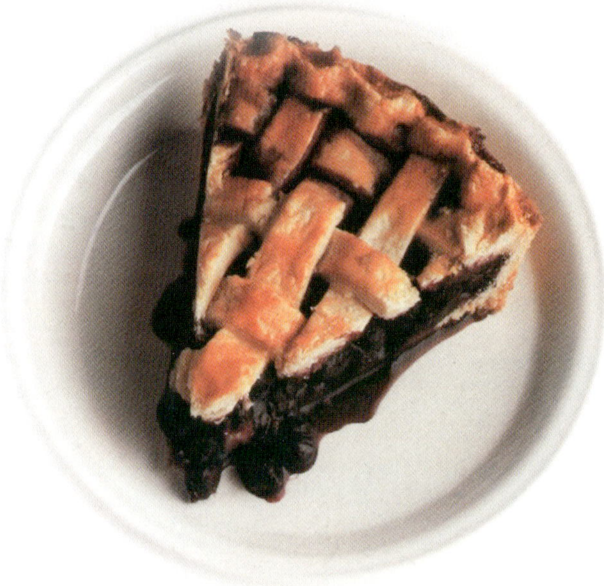